CONTEMPORARY
TAIWANESE
WOMEN WRITERS

CONTEMPORARY TAIWANESE WOMEN WRITERS

An Anthology

EDITED BY

Jonathan Stalling, Lin Tai-man, and Yanwing Leung

Foreword by Pi-twan Huang

A joint project by Cambria Press and
The Taipei Chinese Center, PEN International
in cooperation with Taiwan Academy at TECRO
and Ministry of Culture, Republic of China (Taiwan)

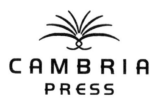

CAMBRIA
PRESS

Amherst, New York

Requests for permission should be directed to
permissions@cambriapress.com, or mailed to:
Cambria Press
100 Corporate Parkway, Suite 128
Amherst, New York 14226, USA

Cover Image: Photo provided by/ Legend Lin Dance Theatre; Photographer/ CHIN,
CHENG-TSAI; Title of work/ *The Eternal Tides*; Dancer/ WU, MING-CHING.

Library of Congress Cataloging-in-Publication Data

Names: Stalling, Jonathan, editor. | Lin, Daiman, 1962- editor. |
Leung, Yan-wing, editor.

Title: Contemporary Taiwanese women writers : an anthology /
edited by Jonathan Stalling, Lin Tai-Man, and Yanwing Leung.

Description: New York : Cambria Press, 2018.

Identifiers: LCCN 2017057953 |

ISBN 9781604979558

Subjects: LCSH: Chinese literature--Taiwan--21st century. |
Chinese literature--Women authors--21st century. |
Chinese literature--21st century--Translations into English.

Classification: LCC PL3031.T32 C66 2018 |
DDC 895.108/092870951249--dc23
LC record available at https://lccn.loc.gov/2017057953

TABLE OF CONTENTS

Foreword
Pi-twan Huang 黃碧端 vii

Introduction: From Taiwan: Some of the Richest Sinophone
Literature
Jonathan Stalling 1

Chapter 1: Wedding Date
Ping Lu 平路 5

Chapter 2: The Story of Hsiao-Pi
Chu T'ien-wen 朱天文 25

Chapter 3: The Party Girl
Lin Tai-man 林黛嫚 37

Chapter 4: Taipei Train Station
Tsai Su-fen 蔡素芬 59

Chapter 5: The Travels and Lover of a Junior High Girl
Chung Wenyin 鍾文音 69

Chapter 6: Baby, My Dear
Marula Liu 劉梓潔 83

Chapter 7: No Time to Grow Up
Su Wei-chen 蘇偉貞 105

Chapter 8: A Place of One's Own
Yuan Chiung-chiung 袁瓊瓊 117

Chapter 9: Seed of the Rape Plant
Liao Hui-ying 廖輝英 139

Chapter 10: The Devil in a Chastity Belt
Li Ang 李昂 167

Chapter 11: The Fish
       Chen Jo-hsi 陳若曦 201

About the Editors 213

FOREWORD

Pi-twan Huang 黃碧端

As a devoted chapter of PEN International, Taipei Chinese PEN has been promoting modern Taiwanese literature to an international readership since 1972 via its flagship journal *A Quarterly Journal of Contemporary Chinese Literature from Taiwan.*

This is a daunting task with far-reaching implications, as Chinese is one of the oldest languages of the world and as such has accumulated an embarrassment of riches of literary gems. Following the rise of Communist China, literary creation was subjected to restrictive guidelines, forcing the exodus of literati in 1949 with the retreat of the Nationalist government to Taiwan. These newcomers injected new blood into the diverse local culture, preserving a tradition of excellence in literature written in Chinese.

In recent years, China's open-door policy has fueled a rapid growth of literary assets and achievements, while Taiwan sustains her role as a bastion of Chinese traditions in literature. The Taipei Chinese PEN is proud to continue, for nearly half a century, introducing excellent Taiwanese literature written in Chinese and appearing in high-quality English translation to a world readership.

Women writers have always played a significant role in literary Taiwan. I need to thank Lin Tai-man especially. Lin is a professor of literature and a seasoned literary editor. She carefully combed a huge collection of works to select the eleven worthy pieces for the present volume. The original translation was edited by Professor Yanwing Leung, Chief Editor of the Taipei Chinese PEN *Quarterly.* I also thank Jack Kuei, Director of the Taiwan Academy in Washington, D.C., for initiating the partnership between Taipei Chinese PEN and Cambria Press, leading to the publication of the present volume in the United States for an English-speaking audience.

Credit also goes to Jonathan Stalling for his generous support and assistance throughout. I sincerely hope that this is only the beautiful beginning of a long and fruitful relationship.

Pi-twan Huang 黃碧端
President, Taipei Chinese PEN

CONTEMPORARY TAIWANESE WOMEN WRITERS

FROM TAIWAN: SOME OF THE RICHEST SINOPHONE LITERATURE

Jonathan Stalling

Anthologies, like conversations, are often an uneven business. Some conversations emerge as procedural, habitual, run-of-the mill occasions passing by like a daily commute, a blurred periphery speeding unremarkably into the oblivion of time. Others appear as an unexpectedly sublime sunset; still others fall upon us like a traffic accident, unassimilable, numbing. Yet the conversations in this collection are unlike other encounters—each arrives from a singular sentience, a vocative language connecting one to another, revealing experiences different from and yet relatable to any reader's own.

As we begin the anthology, we find ourselves in the shoes of Hsu Tsui-hsuan in Lin Tai-man's story "The Party Girl" as a gifted storyteller relays her tale to the narrator in the hopes that it may help her navigate the fraught waters of class, sex, and perhaps even love itself:

> "It'll take a while to tell my whole story. I'll go into a lot of detail, you know, and tell it slowly. But you don't have anything better to do at the moment anyway, am I right? So, I'll just talk and you listen. Please don't interrupt me, or I'll lose the thread of what I'm saying. If you have any questions, please wait until I'm finished. When I first saw you at that reception today, I figured you were the same kind of person I am. So I think my personal experiences might be useful to you. Should I be mistaken about this, and you're after all a different person from me, it doesn't matter, either. Just listen to it as you'd listen to a story, 'cause it's an interesting story that I've got to tell."

In a sense, each story unfolds like this, in narratives spanning adolescence, marriage, and motherhood as well as sex, politics, and economics on many different scales—some appear as snapshots of lives in transition, others reveal whole lives as time-lapse images, while a few implode into the stillness of a single bottomless moment. Individually, each story expresses its own varied, expansively heterogeneous narrative, yet, taken as a whole, we discover a pointedly gendered exploration of modern Taiwan in works that span more than four decades.

A Pacific island of roughly 14,400 square miles, Taiwan lies just over a hundred miles off China's southeast shoreline and seven hundred miles south of Japan. It has been a contested cultural space between its original aboriginal inhabitants (Taiyals and Vonums), and then among many generations of Chinese immigrants as well as waves of Dutch, Spanish, and Japanese colonial inhabitants, all of which provides the backdrop for some of the richest Sinophone literature in the world. Unfixed, vibrant, and deeply engaged with a sense of place, Taiwanese writers—from the experimental poetry pioneer Hsia Yu to younger multimedia poets like Ye Mimi to powerhouse authors like Li Ang and Chu T'ien-wen—are continually pushing the boundaries of the possible and unlocking new directions for Sinophone literature in the twenty-first century.

With this first American anthology of contemporary Taiwanese women writers in decades, the editors hope to expose English readers to the widest possible range of voices, styles, and textures of contemporary Taiwanese writers. In Ping Lu's "Wedding Date," we meet a wheelchair-bound mother who seems to get younger by the day as her filial daughter prematurely ages. A talented writer in her youth, the protagonist's imagination imbues a possible romance with an intimacy that seems so real it almost becomes so, despite piling signs to the contrary. In "The Story of Hsiao-Pi," by Newman Prize–winning author Chu T'ien-wen, the narrator lovingly examines the life of a troubled village boy, who builds an unexpected future upon the fierce if complicated love of his mother and step-father. Then Taiwan itself becomes the protagonist in Tsai Su-fen's "Taipei Train Station," where the station serves as an aperture through which numerous lives pass, if only briefly, into view before emerging into the boundless possibilities of the city.

Chung Wenyin recalls her first steps into literature and love through her story "The Travels and Lover of a Junior High Girl," an adventure that explores the evolving ideas of love and the eros of art, and the open-ended possibilities of life itself. After being told by an amateur psychic that her not-yet-conceived son is following her around, waiting for his time to enter the world, the narrator of Marula Liu's story "Baby, My Dear" begins to search for his father. Su Wei-chen, however, enters the traumatic space of a mother losing her daughter to leukemia in "No Time to Grow Up," asking if children who die so young have had enough time to even know they are alive. Yuan Chiung-chiung traces the dynamic and transformative process of divorce, reinvention, and love through the story "A Place of One's Own," while Liao Hui-ying opens a window into class identity, fate, motherhood, and, ultimately, love in the context of an arranged marriage in "Seed of the Rape Plant." Li Ang offers a tale of Taiwanese oppositional politics, personal sacrifice, and unrequited love in "The Devil in a Chastity Belt." Chen Jo-hsi draws the collection to a close with a poignant vignette exposing the point where international politics and the dinner table meet, somewhere between the imagination and anticipation and the machinations of political power in her story "The Fish."

Regarding a few practical matters—throughout the anthology we have retained the original currency amounts in the New Taiwan Dollar, colloquially referred to as "a dollar." From the 1960s to about 1985, one US Dollar was worth approximately thirty to forty NT Dollars. Also, readers who are more familiar with Pinyin, the Chinese Romanization system used in mainland China, the Romanization of Taiwan names and places may seem strange at first glance. This is because many Taiwanese writers use a combination of Romanization systems (including a simplified version of Wade-Giles and Tongyong Pinyin, among others). From a practical standpoint, students do not learn a single Romanization system in Taiwan, so there is little reason to standardize name spellings, yet when read at a deeper level, the uniqueness of Taiwanese orthography—from its use of traditional/complex Chinese characters to its unfixed systems of Romanization—reveals a deep connection between Taiwan and its multifaceted linguistic history. Taken as a whole, Taiwan literature, like its complex writing systems, exists in the present as a rich palimpsest of the cultural contact points, overlapping languages, peoples, and histories that have paved the way for one of the most vibrant literary scenes in the Sinosphere and the world beyond.

CHAPTER 1

WEDDING DATE

婚期

Ping Lu 平路

(Translated by Sylvia Li-chun Lin 林麗君)

My first question was: Who copied the thought in my head without my permission?

My second question was: When the thought grew more powerful, could its mere conception be considered a crime?

I was wandering about at the scene, looking for an answer, until you took my arm and led me here.

1

When you were a child, you must have played with fire.

You must have savored the experience: The match burns shorter and shorter in your fingers and the painful burning sensation in your nerve endings forces you to drop it, but for an instant you are reluctant to see the light go out.

During the Ghost Festival in the seventh month, you've watched the sacrificial paper curl up in the flames, the blackened paper with crimson edges roiling with the seductive tongues of fire in an iron brazier. Squatting there, I felt the ground start to heat up. Even when my face was burning red and my feet had turned numb, I was still poking and looking, searching for paper that had not yet turned to ashes...

"Namah Amitabha, tathagata..." Paper figurines were lowered into the fire amid the chanting of the Reincarnation Mantra, as if conducting a dialogue between the land of the living and the nether world. "Ami patuta, vikarati, Ami patuta, vikarata..." *Burned to ashes*, I thought, *was one way to end—to end the feelings of gratitude and resentment that were impossible to disentangle.*

2

You're too conscientious. It's only a case, but you've spared no effort, even trying to learn about my past. With a wry smile I look at an old manuscript of mine that you hold in your hands, a brief short story called "Love Nest."

After counting the pages of the photocopied manuscript, you put one copy in your file folder and hand the other to me.

The words I've written now seem unfamiliar.

It's a simple story: A man directs a monologue at a house he has designed. He thinks about the past, looking very guilty, because,

> Their living conditions have never been ideal: A duplex crammed into a noisy alley; they have to climb three flights of filthy stairs in the dark to get to a small apartment made of construction materials that are showing their age.

The reason he blames himself also has something to do with his job:

> ...as an employee of a construction company, over the past few years, he has drawn up many floor plans for clients and has supervised workers in putting up model homes. His salary isn't bad, but he is unable to give his wife a house he has personally designed.

This time, he finally has a chance:

> ...according to the blueprint, the most unique feature of the new house is the rhomboid-shaped skylight. On sunny days, bright light splashes on the floor from the skylight, like sparkles reflecting off a crystal chandelier. On wet days, raindrops shatter against the glass. He can visualize, during the endless days that follow, the look in his wife's eyes as she loses herself in the sound of the rain.

> He doesn't like phony, gaudy colors. In his striving for an ingenious touch, the ground floor of his house is encircled by a white porch. In the cool summer evening breezes, he imagines, his wife can sit in a rocking chair on the porch, as watery moonlight trickles down the fair skin on the down-covered nape of her neck...

"The writing is tight and refined." Waving the file folder in your hand, you look at me somewhat incredulously, trying to discover something in my dull expression. Of course, what interests you most is the surprise ending:

> Now he looks up at his wife, whose expression shows no sign of resentment. The woman in the picture frame is staring at him— watching him consign the newly built house to flames.

At that moment, I, too, am surprised. Flames? Burned up in a fire? How could I have known so long ago what the ending would be like?

3

That was perhaps my most well crafted work.

In my younger days, as a college graduate majoring in Chinese, I showed some literary promise. It was that promise that was eaten away by years of working at a desk.

Even now, I can still create invisible details in my imagination. For instance, standing in the barely hundred-square-foot room I share with my mother, my eyes will, as if transforming the rotten into something magical, strip off the old wallpaper and replace it with heavy woven curtains. A breeze blows past, sending the white satin tassels fluttering out the window... Ah, how lithe and lively they are!

I have always enjoyed this kind of game. When I come to a scenic spot, I wistfully imagine that someday I will return with my beloved and walk on the beach one more time. As a matter of fact, several years ago, even though I didn't have a suitable partner, I mapped out an itinerary for my round-island honeymoon. The little inn at Golden Sand Bay, located on the tip of the cape, would be our first stop.

I never tire of such games. I even subscribe to bridal magazines from abroad. I spend a great deal of time studying trends in wedding gowns, keeping an eye out for new styles and tailoring, as if I'll be next. Sometimes in my imagination, I even decorate the site of my wedding ceremony. A small church will do; I prefer the atmosphere of a church even though I'm not a believer. I've noticed in other people's weddings an arch decorated with roses and an aisle covered with rose petals. Red roses represent love. The train of the bride's gown follows her down the aisle, through the door that leads to happiness.

What about music? Would the organ in the church work? The song "We've Only Just Begun." A long, long journey has just begun...how romantic!

I'm forever pondering the finer points of the dress: a sweetheart neckline, a drop waist to lengthen the upper body and create a statuesque illusion, bouffant sleeves with georgette lace from the elbow down. As for the skirt, years ago I settled on one decorated with heart-shaped ruffles and white satin rosettes. What about a hat? I prefer a broad-brimmed hat with a big bow that flutters to the rhythm of the wedding march. Yet a broad brim might obscure the graceful shoulder line... I saw enough dress patterns as a little girl to be quite sure of the details. And it was precisely because of my ability to handle details that, standing before a full-length mirror, I could witness the flowing lace consumed in a raging fire, without being present at the scene. The flammable satin train would add fuel to the fire. What a mesmerizing, soul-stirring picture that is!

I can picture a bride, totally intoxicated by happiness only a moment before, running out of the dressing room, holding her long skirt as she flees in panic...

Amid the frenzied footsteps, decorative beads loosened from the dress roll across the floor, reflecting a strange luster in the flames. In the next instant, the shine fades completely in the intense heat, and they look like Buddha relics emerging from a crematorium... Apathetically, I conjure up the scene of destruction after the fire. I am well aware that there is a cruel side to my nature.

Undeniably cruel! For a long time, I've been yearning for a way to end this miserable situation.

Last month a fire broke out in our building. In the middle of the night, someone banged frantically on my door. I jumped out of bed, opened the door a crack and looked into the hallway, where people were running. "Use the rear exit, not the front!" Voices shouting noisily. For me it was a nightmare come true. I've always been fearful that our elevator would be out of service. Would I be able to pick up my mother and put her in a wheelchair, and, if so, could the wheelchair negotiate the rusty emergency stairs? From where she lay in bed, my mother looked all around with darting eyes; she was already struggling to get up, her thin arms outstretched. I bent down, straining to hoist her onto my back. Her legs virtually useless, she grabbed hold of me tightly. I could barely breathe with her on my back. How could I possibly make my way down that narrow stairwell, which was barely wide enough for one person?

Calling upon all my strength, I carried her to the head of the stairs. The sounds of our neighbors were distant; they'd probably all made it safely to ground level. I smelled whiffs of her greasy hair oil, sensed the rancid odor of her body heat, and detected the rotten stench in her mouth. Was a fire raging? Maybe it was out already; maybe it was just a silly prank. At that instant, a wicked idea suddenly formed in my mind: What if I were to pry loose her fingers and let her tumble down the stairs? When people found a paralyzed old woman lying in a pool of blood, her daughter wailing beside her (I could put on a very convincing act), no one would show any surprise, since losing one's footing during a fire was a common accident.

Many years ago, hadn't Mother herself made up a similarly outlandish story?

As I stood there, I was already aware that fires can kindle incredibly evil ideas in people's minds. And, more importantly, they are a perfect means to eliminate evidence, for what remains is nothing but ashes.

But it was only a fleeting thought. The next day, I was once again sitting across from Mother, watching her gleefully gnaw on a fish head as strange gurgling sounds emerged from her throat. Then she casually spit the bones all over the table for me to pick up. Now that she spent her days in a wheelchair, something unusual was happening —she apparently enjoyed food more than I, her appetite far better than mine. At dinnertime, as I watched her eat with such gusto, I felt the same resentment I'd experienced in my childhood. I'd hated her for turning me into a laughingstock at school with uniforms she patched together with remnants from her clients... When I cried and refused to go to school, she beat me again and again with her yardstick.

Was it because I couldn't fight back? I thought my childhood wounds had healed, but they actually followed me like a shadow, growing bigger and bigger as I did.

Then she'd put down her chopsticks and smack her lips. She always let out a booming belch, so loud that, even with no one else around, I felt embarrassed for her. Her belches were getting louder every year, all for my sake, I'm sure. Since she was so limited in what she could do, she needed something to force me to take note of her existence.

A belch and several huge yawns a couple of hours later—these were the main events in Mother's life. We hardly ever talked. To be more precise, I seldom gave her a chance to talk to me, a sort of passive resistance. Besides that, I exacted limited revenge in every possible way, however small. For instance, I knew she was dying for some fresh air, and I could have taken her out to eat in her wheelchair. But I didn't. I'd rather order food to go. It was just too much trouble going up and down the stairs, I told myself. I'd rather stand at a food stall every evening and wait for the woman to bag two boxes of rice and gravy.

"Miss, wouldn't you like to try something different?" she asked, with the best of intentions. No, I shook my head impassively, waiting for her to fill the box with half a braised fish and a ladleful of hollow greens.

"You folks sure live simply, the same thing every day," the woman muttered.

Inwardly, I smiled, a bitter smile... If there were a choice, who would opt for a life of monotony? Who would reject one filled with brightness?

The first time I saw Chen-wei, I was sitting in a dark corner in a coffee shop when he opened the glass door and walked in, the light at his back. The sunshine from trees on the sidewalk lingered on his face. At that instant, I felt my cheeks burn and my heartbeat quicken for no apparent reason...

Given his advantageous circumstances, Chen-wei could never under-stand the value of pulling someone out of darkness, just as he could never comprehend what it was like to live a life devoid of hope.

4

For many years, I sank deeper and deeper into the quagmire of a life so rigidly disciplined it was virtually stagnant. It took a great deal of effort just to open my eyes in the morning.

I wasn't sick, just lethargic, lacking vitality. Before I took a single step forward, the power of darkness enveloped me.

No wonder I was putting on weight, gaining extra inches of fat. Not only was my waist thicker, but so was my neck. The cuffs of my short-sleeved shirts were so tight there was no room for movement. Most surprising of all was that my shoes were getting a half-size larger each year.

My mother seemed to be the only one who could turn back the clock. Strangely, she stopped aging after her stroke. As she pushed herself around the apartment in her wheelchair, the black spots on her face gradually disappeared, revealing a glow unseen before.

In my dreams, Mother, who slept next to me, was clearly younger than I. She looked even younger than during my early years when she slumped behind her sewing machine. When I woke up, I entertained the bitter thought that I, her daughter, was the one who was growing old, thanks to her.

I listened to her cough, spit, and clear her throat every night, listened to her lift herself out of bed and into her creaky wheelchair, listened to her hoist herself out of the wheelchair onto the toilet. Then came the sounds of her tugging at toilet paper, flushing the toilet, straining with her arms to transport herself back onto the wheelchair (a few drops of urine would always be left behind on the toilet seat)... Just being entangled in my mother's life was enough to cause me to lose interest in everything else. Yes, I've lost a lot during these years: My fertility was rapidly disappearing (I was already thirty-eight years old), and my senses were growing dull. When I reread my earlier writings, I wondered if they were really mine. Gradually, I found it hard to believe that I'd once woven stories with words.

During periods of depression, just getting through the day was nearly impossible... I had to cajole myself just to go on living. As for Mother, she sang songs behind my back from the old days, like a little girl. When I walked in on her, she abruptly stopped singing, covering her mouth as if she'd done something wrong.

Mother knew only that I didn't like loud noises, so I told her that, ever since I was a little girl, I'd had all I could take of the wearisome sound of her sewing machine.

She looked up at me with an expression like that of a wounded animal. From then on, whenever I was home, she tried hard not to make any noise. She didn't even dare turn on the TV before I left for work.

Were the two of us, mother and daughter, competing silently for something? If she won, I would have to lose.

The age spots on Mother's face were getting lighter and lighter, approaching invisibility. When I looked at myself in the mirror, I found a black spot the size of a coin above my left cheekbone.

Many evenings, as I lay in bed, I knew she was still awake, staring at me in the dark, like a cat waiting for the right time to pounce.

At the same time, I felt my own body sink little by little, submerge inch by inch.

I was desperate for a way out, and some sort of sudden change seemed to be my only hope. When I met Chen-wei, I thought I'd found that way out, like crawling forward on the ground and suddenly seeing a glimmer of light at the end of the tunnel...

For happy people, I guess, a stirring sensation only adds something extra to an already contented life. But for someone like me, this sensation was all the compensation I needed; my life now had the promise I longed for.

During those days, I saw mockery in my mother's eyes. She must have intuited a change in my circumstances (I sometimes came home late, but not that late, shortly after dinner). She'd be in her wheelchair, waiting for me, an unconcealed sinister smile on her face. In reality, Mother knew all along (How did she know?); there were all those curses she'd hurled at me when I was a child—back then, sitting at her sewing machine, she'd curse over and over again: "Big hands and big feet, such an unlucky girl! You won't be filial enough to make my grave clothes, so don't expect me to look happily at you in a bridal gown."

5

For years, I enjoyed reading real estate advertisements, fingering the little squares one by one until I settled on one in a lovely style I liked. Then I'd imagine myself living in that house, with several rooms needing to be decorated. I'd pick out a wallpaper design and a color for the window drapes, then I'd choose the furniture, tablecloth, sheets... Like assembling Legos, I'd sketch out a picture of home in my head.

Maybe that's why I wrote the short story called "Love Nest" years ago. Placing myself in the imagined house, I saw the wind billowing the window drapes inward, with the soft yellow plissé crepe stroking my face. Ruffles of a similar color brought the drapes all the way to the floor.

When I was a little girl, bolts of fabric brought over by customers were piled up around Mother's sewing machine, but she never allowed me to touch them, saying, "What will we do if you soil them?" So I sat there, using my imagination to give each piece of colorful cloth a design chosen from her dress pattern books...

The wall behind the sewing machine was pasted with pictures cut out from magazines. All of lovely Japanese women in Western-style one- or two-piece dresses decorated with big buttons, styles popular among doctors' wives in town but of no relevance to me. Except for one, the picture of a wedding gown, a bouffant skirt that barely reached the knees, plus a pair of elbow-length white gloves.

It was probably a popular style for wedding gowns in those days. I used to touch that picture and imagine what the georgette (especially the white lace across the chest) would feel like.

"You weren't born to wear that kind of dress!" Mother would say with a sneer when she saw me daydreaming.

I'd sulk and imagine myself striking a match then burning the stack of fabric next to her machine to ashes, wondering if it would give off a caustic odor. Mother often did that, waving a lit match over a piece of cloth and asking the customer to sniff while she told them whether or not they'd bought fake wool.

Mother once told me with great earnestness that my father had been a firefighter who'd died in a disastrous fire.

I never really believed her, because the word "Unknown" was what it said in the column for "Father" on my ID card.

A neighbor woman once whispered to me that a handsome young man had been helping out in the shop, but took off when the owner's belly began to swell. A fire of unknown origin broke out the day he left, but was extinguished before it spread. The woman next door was the one who poured the first basin of water on it.

Was it the fire that gave Mother the idea of "firefighter"?

The neighbor woman was clearly more believable. Mother made a slip of the tongue once when she was scolding me for not wanting to learn dressmaking and for my clumsy peddling of the sewing machine, causing it to jam.

It just slipped out: "You're just like that drop-dead good-for-nothing, who broke a needle every time he pedaled the machine!"

Was Mother still thinking about him? Except for that one slip of the tongue, I never got another clue out of her.

Maybe that's where Mother and I were alike; we were both strong-willed. In her mind, the man would be burned to ashes once he left her.

There is no place for compromise in the realm of love; it's either a raging fire or there isn't even a spark...

Before Chen-wei, I'd met other men, even some who were longing for marriage, just like me. And there were always eager colleagues who enjoyed being matchmakers; they urged me not to be too picky. I wasn't young anymore, so why be so choosy? But I often found myself losing patience after the first date. It was nauseating to discover the flaws in these men, who picked their noses, smacked their lips, clinked their knives and forks, scraped their plates clean, or let a thin thread of sticky saliva ooze from between their lips. I'd rejected every one of them, not giving them a second chance.

"You stubborn little brat!" That's what Mother used to say about me.

Just before Chen-wei showed up in my life, I had a dream in which the shadow of a man with a blurred face reached out for my hand. In my dream I understood that he wanted to take me with him, step by step. When I touched his hand, a cool sensation like soft sand running through my palm made this a peaceful, sweet dream, something I seldom enjoyed.

When Chen-wei pushed open the door and walked into the coffee shop, I was sitting in a dark corner, drifting into a kind of trance. Was that because of the dream, or had I just been lonely too long? I fixed my gaze on Chen-wei's face: I'd waited so long, but it was him, the man with the blurred face in my dream.

So we started seeing each other. For me, those were days of endless anticipation (or maybe I should say supplication). We always went out after work, and he always ordered the daily special. He'd smile politely and begin with some small-talk ("It's been getting hot again the past few days," or "I'm busy at work, always busy"), then leisurely pick up his knife and fork, cut his food into tiny pieces, and chew them slowly, his eyes cast down, as if I didn't exist in his world, even though I was sitting across from him.

While those might be called dates, sometimes I suspected that he just wanted a leisurely meal after work. After dinner, he'd put me in a taxi and say he'd see me next week.

After much time had passed (actually I'd spent a long time standing in front of my dressing mirror), I yearned for him to see something attractive in my plain face. (Once, when my supervisor was in good mood, he told me that it took a long time to discover the tender beauty of my face.) I put on some newly bought lipstick and learned to walk in high heels (after nearly spraining my ankle), all because of my feelings for a man...

During the months we were together, I desperately wanted to tell Chen-wei how I felt about him, but was afraid he'd be frightened away by an open declaration. If so, then I'd be like a free-falling object, plunging straight back into that previous changeless, deadened existence...

Then again, it would have brought me indescribable happiness to leave the door open just a crack and learn that he liked me, even a little.

I believed...if I'd been given a little time and the promise of a life together, that he'd have begun to understand me as he sat in a house I'd decorated, at a table covered with a tablecloth I'd carefully chosen, eating a meal I'd cooked for him. And someday, he might actually have come to love me, finding it hard to ever leave me.

But he never gave me the chance.

6

Chen-wei could not understand the significance of pulling someone out of the muck.

My life was fulfilled after I met Chen-wei. I didn't see him often, but I roamed the field of my exquisitely imagined world, reluctant to leave it.

I made repeated trips to department stores, where I visited the bedroom section so I could decorate the bedroom of my imagination. My favorite bedspread was one with tiny flowers sprinkled among entangled vines. Sheets? I chose a similar design with tiny flowers, but without the vines, trying to imagine the effect created by the slight difference.

I never dared to envision other aspects, such as the look of a bed sheet crumpled by two bodies.

When we met, Chen-wei always sat rigidly across the table from me. He kept his arms close to his sides when he wasn't using his knife and fork. It was as if there were an invisible barrier, one he never had the courage to cross over.

Ever since childhood, I've had a phobia about bodily contact. When sleeping with Mother, I was always fearful of her breath blowing into my face; it gave me a clammy, unclean feeling. Yet for years I've had to lift Mother into a bathtub once a week, watching her breasts that sagged to her navel begin to float as if losing weight, and her gray pubic hair spread out in the nourishing warm water.

After meeting Chen-wei, I spent more time sitting in the tub, scrubbing my body with a brush made of a dried loofah gourd, cleaning my concave belly button, my damp armpits, and the creases in the lips of my vulva. Soaking in the water, I'd rinse and scrub my body with water from the hand-held shower, never tiring of the cleansing process. I'd unconsciously repeat the same motions, over and over, maybe because I was afraid I might carry some sort of bad odor.

Sometimes I'd ask myself why I tried to make my body so clean. What kind of rite was I preparing for?

Chen-wei didn't even intend to hold my hand.

Sitting across from me at the table, waiting for our food to be served, he'd say half-heartedly: "It absolutely poured today. It's rained a lot lately, I wonder why."

He didn't expect an answer.

But I liked to hear the sound of his voice, which, like melodious raindrops, allowed me to linger in my imagined house, where the window curtains fluttered in the damp air to reveal an embroidered gauze screen, and beads of water splattered against the windowpane... Chen-wei said something, but I couldn't make it out. We lived in separate, self-contained worlds. He talked to me without waiting for a response. He didn't even look into my eyes when he talked, as if he were afraid he might encounter some carelessly divulged secrets...

I often felt giddy as I sat across from him. It was like slowly waking up after soaking in a tub. The ceiling seemed to have turned. Had I fallen asleep?

Afraid he might detect a lack of interest, I nervously sat up straight.

It was at our usual restaurant, the one called "Family," where he calmly brought up the idea. He finished his soup and dabbed his face with a paper napkin before he casually said: "If you have no objection, why don't we take out a marriage license to fulfill our family's wishes and put our parents at ease?"

Was he proposing? Was he actually proposing to me? Had he begun to like me? Had he decided he wanted to live with me? It was so sudden; there was no warning. In disbelief, I steadied myself by holding onto the table. At that instant, a vague happiness rippled through my heart.

Without waiting for my answer, he continued: "We don't have to change our lifestyles. You can keep living where you are. Marriage," he paused, "for modern people, is often just a formality."

I was momentarily at a loss for words.

After a long silence, I could only think of one thing. Imitating his tone, I spoke, haltingly, as if pleading with him: "Wedding pictures, eh, something we have to do, no?"

Then I looked up to see a solemn expression on his face.

"As a commemoration, that's fine. If that's what you want, we can do that," he finally said unemotionally.

7

As the wedding date neared (the date we'd agreed upon to go to the courthouse), we saw each other less and less.

Chen-wei, as it turned out, was busier than ever at work. Except for meeting him at a restaurant, where we silently shared a meal, I was left to take care of the wedding dress.

I suddenly realized that all along I'd pictured no one else but me, wearing a bridal veil in my repeated creations of a wedding scene.

At a boutique on Chung-shan North Road, I was surprised to find a wedding gown that perfectly fit the final design, after many revisions in my mind: sweetheart neckline, drop waist, and a long bouffant skirt that fell to the floor, with heart-shaped ruffles and white satin bow rosettes... Standing in front of the dressing mirror, I looked at myself from every angle, at my slender figure with a waist made slim by a corset. In the mirror...it was a dream come true.

I recalled a day before I'd met Chen-wei, when I went into a tourist hotel to use their clean bathroom. As I came out of the ladies' room, a golden light from a skylight gilded the scene of a couple in wedding attire. Their slightly upturned faces looked soft and bright under the reflected light. If there was truly something called happiness in this world, I believed that was it.

I decided to insert myself into the brightness of that day.

The more anxious I grew over gains and losses, the harder I tried to pretend that nothing was wrong, so Mother wouldn't detect any change.

In the meantime, I still couldn't muster the courage to ask Chen-wei to do more.

As I think back, I realize he was probably unconvinced that all I'd wanted was for him to stand beside me (actually, every time he looked at me, there was guilt in his eyes).

I went to a wedding photo studio every day to flip through the bulky photo albums they used to attract customers. There were always trivial details that required a decision.

After I'd been there several times, I noticed a spiral staircase in the shape of a chimney. One afternoon, as I was walking down the steps, I nearly tripped on the skirt, which was too long for me (it was later altered to fit my height). When I first tried on the wedding gown, even in high heels borrowed from the boutique, I had to stand on tiptoes to avoid stepping on the hem.

Every time it was me, only me, going over to alter the gown, to choose the shoes, to pick out matching earrings, to try on the dress, again and again, then return a third time for alterations... It was as if I were playing house alone.

Chen-wei's presence was required for the dress rehearsal. Now, when I think back, it might have been a bad decision, if, indeed, there had been a mistake at all.

After he entered the photo studio at the agreed time, he lowered his eyes when he saw my powdered face, but not before I caught the glint of fright in his expression.

He closed his eyes as if enduring torture while the make-up artist powdered his face and penciled his eyebrows. The director told him to hold my hands and look at me with tenderness and love. I could tell he complied with reluctance.

That afternoon, we went outside to photograph some alfresco scenes. As we followed behind the photography equipment balanced on the shoulders of people who told us where to stand and what to do, Chen-wei was looking increasingly impatient. He kept raising his eyebrows, as if trying very hard to control himself. I wished he'd turn to look at me, at my pleading eyes.

Amid shrill, ear-splitting automobile horns, a spot was found on the safety island, which would produce a picture of lush green lawns. The photographer mumbled that these shots were guaranteed to look European. In the bright sunlight, I wore my hair in braids and was holding a lovely little parasol. A pair of thin gold-rimmed glasses was perched on Chen-wei's nose; he was wearing a glittery cummerbund around his waist and a pleated tuxedo shirt.

Sweat stained his back as he was photographed under the blazing sun. He wasn't short, but his legs looked stocky with that wide cummerbund around his waist.

I realized at that moment that I should have found a better style for him.

Holding a mirror in one hand while the make-up artist re-powdered my face, I kept looking over at Chen-wei with mounting concern. The photographer was gesturing and instructing him how to pose.

Suddenly, a voice—someone's voice—was raised. I quickly put down the mirror and looked over, only to see an agitated expression I'd never seen before on Chen-wei's face, as if he were waging one last struggle with himself.

"Phony!" I heard him shout as he tore at the cummerbund around his waist.

Tossing away that gaudy piece of cloth and loosening his bow tie, he walked off, faster and faster, and soon he had made it to the other side of the safety island. He crossed the street and started running down the sidewalk...

I just stared as he disappeared at the first intersection.

Afterward, he didn't come to see me again, not even a phone call.

A few days later, the manager of the photo studio told me the balance had been paid in full.

Then someone relayed a message from Chen-wei, who said he was very sorry. Of course I knew it was all over between us when he said that. There had been no solid ground to begin with, and now, after this, it was all over.

The most ridiculous thing was, the store delivered an enlarged, framed studio wedding photo to the flat I shared with my mother. Fastened with a red satin ribbon, it had been placed on my bed, like a gift of great joy.

While I was still at work, my silent mother, with her squinting eyes, had already seen through this farce, one that needed no explanation from me.

In fact, she'd known all along. It was that curse she'd hurled at me all over again: How could I expect to ever have that kind of good fortune?

Looking at the mocking smile on the photograph, I was reminded of an incident from my childhood: After a quarrel with Mother, I peeled off a swatch of cloth from her dress pattern book and pasted it onto another page. She went ahead and made the dress, unaware that it was the wrong style and size for her customer. As a result, she locked me up in the house and beat me with her yardstick.

"Wrong, wrong, wrong…" I muttered over and over as I knelt on the cold cement floor.

Now, facing the enlarged wedding photo, I heard my own voice: When it's wrong, there's no chance of ever turning back.

8

Happiness is actually very fragile. It can turn to ashes at any moment, don't you think?

I moved quietly on the spiral staircase, followed by a breeze in the wake of my movement. A candle held high in my hand illuminated newlyweds in the picture frames.

In the shadowy darkness, I sensed my mother's pinched nasal voice, her somniloquy interspersed with curses. My sweaty palms were clammy; had she caught up with me? The air was getting hotter and dryer...

I imagined myself in a floor-length bouffant skirt with white satin rosettes, fleeing in panic amid a crowd. In the steamy, thick smoke, would you reach out to me as you pass? You should help a woman who has tripped and fallen.

I lit a match and touched it to the wedding photos. The frames caught on fire; acrylic frames writhing in the intense heat, mannequins toppling backward, and hanging curtains gave off an odorous stench...pairs of newlyweds burned into charred holes; this is the funeral I arranged for happiness.

You probably won't believe me, because it's such a flimsy excuse: How could an erroneously delivered wedding photo become the cause of arson?

But you ought to know that there is a kind of longing that is like stretching your neck to seek out the light. This longing always burns most brightly in the dark, when there is no one around.

> * From Ping Lu's 平路 *Pai-ling Chien* «百齡箋» (*One-hundred-year-old Note*) (Taipei: Unitas Publishing, 1998). This translation won the twelfth Liang Shih-chiu Awards for Chinese-to-English Translation.

Chapter 2

The Story of Hsiao-Pi

小畢的故事

Chu T'ien-wen 朱天文

(Translated by David van der Peet 范德培)

Hsiao-Pi was my classmate in elementary school. His family was our next-door neighbor, having lived in the village over ten years when we moved there. I still remember the first time I saw Hsiao-Pi. It was on the day we moved in. I was busy arranging flowerpots in the yard, lining them up along the fence, when somebody suddenly called me from across the roses on the other side of the fence. "Hey!" I raised my head to look: ugh, a dark-skinned boy. I walked over, and the boy said, "I know your family name is Chu…" Then he tore a big, shiny green caterpillar apart, right before my eyes. He could not have known that I was not in the least scared of caterpillars. I grabbed some soil and hurled it at him. Seeing that his attempt to scare me had not been successful, he yelled angrily, "Chu's your name, meaning pig! Pig! Hahaha," he said, repeating the word "pig" in Taiwanese to make it sound more insulting. After that, he ran off.

I was assigned to Class A in the fifth grade in elementary school. Our teacher was talking to us from the platform, introducing me to my new classmates and asking us to get along well with each other. At that moment, I saw Hsiao-Pi sitting in the last row at the back of the classroom, stretching a rubber band on his fingers and aiming it toward me. "Pi Chu-chia!" the teacher scolded him sternly. Hsiao-Pi grinned sheepishly and slipped the rubber band up his arm again. Only then could I see that his other arm was covered to the elbow with rubber bands. Rumor had it he'd won all these from the other boys in a popular game. Hsiao-Pi was the forward on the school's dodgeball team. Often he would dash into the classroom, his body giving off an odor that was a strange mixture of sweat and dust. Next he would gulp down a whole bottle of water in no time, rush out again, and leave behind a lingering smell of perspiration.

There were five people in Hsiao-Pi's family. Only later did I find out that Hsiao-Pi's mother had worked in a processing factory in Taoyuan when she was young. There she had fallen in love with her foreman and became pregnant with his child. The foreman was a married man, though, and they had no future. Hsiao-Pi's mother tried to commit suicide by cutting her wrists, but she was rescued and gave birth to Hsiao-Pi. She had to let friends take care of her baby while she found herself a job as a taxi dancer in a nightclub. That job allowed her to pay some of the expenses of bringing up her son. Hsiao-Pi had a rough time of it, and every time his mother visited him she would cry to see him so unhappy. As soon as she had a little bit of money, she rented an apartment together with a fellow taxi dancer, a small place that yet provided all the basic necessities and permitted her to take back her son and live under the same roof with him. In the evenings she would lock the door and go to work.

Uncle Pi already had a wife in mainland China, but they were separated when he fled with the Kuomintang to Taiwan. He had been with a logistics unit ever since the civil war. Uncle Pi was of stocky build with the large hands and feet of a farmer. Being no longer young, he decided to look for a wife to keep him company, and that's where his old friends from Henan Province proved to be very helpful. They asked and looked around, and in the end introduced Hsiao-Pi's mother to Uncle Pi. She was his junior by twenty years. Their first meeting took place in a restaurant. Hsiao-Pi's mother, pale and skinny as she was, must have aroused his pity, for it was as if he felt ashamed for taking advantage of her situation, and afraid of treating her and her son shabbily. Hsiao-Pi's mother asked only for one thing before giving her consent: Uncle Pi had to promise to pay for Hsiao-Pi's expenses until he finished college. The second time they met Uncle Pi proposed to her, bringing presents of betrothal exactly as custom prescribed. Hsiao-Pi's mother did not say anything at the time, but in her heart she was grateful for that.

When they got married, Hsiao-Pi was five years old. When he was seven, a brother was born, and another one a year later. Both his younger brothers were nice kids who did well in school. Mrs. Pi never gave the impression she was particularly happy, but she never seemed particularly unhappy, either. She was always neatly made up, going about her housework silently and efficiently. She would never chat with neighbors, never gossip with them about other people, but always would greet them politely. When Hsiao-Pi had smashed a neighbor's window, or plucked the feather from someone's chicken to make a shuttlecock, Mrs. Pi could be seen standing at the neighbor's doorstep, apologizing in a soft voice, her face flushed before she had even opened her mouth.

Uncle Pi was quite different with his broad, big-boned face and ruddy complexion, his loud voice, and his uproarious laughter. Coming back from work, he would wash himself, move a rattan chair into the yard, and sit down to relax and play with his two sons. They would take turns riding on his feet that were so strong he could raise a boy high into the air with one quick lift. Once up in the air, the younger boy would get scared and start to cry. After being let down, though, he would usually giggle in a silly way. When Mrs. Pi had brought in the laundry, she sometimes stood in the doorway and watched the father and his sons having fun with each other. She would simply stand there with a calm face. She watched for so long and in such an absorbed manner that I often wondered whether she was just staring absent-mindedly, not really watching at all. Around this time of the day, Hsiao-Pi was likely to be still roaming about outside. Mrs. Pi would also smile, which was rare for her. When she did smile, or when she said a few more words than usual, her otherwise skinny and pale cheeks would suddenly glow with the color of peach blossoms. Often when she was standing still for a while in the bright light of day, small pale freckles would appear all over her cheeks and the tip of her nose. Recalling it now, Mrs. Pi's peach-blossom glow looked rather like the sunset clouds that suddenly light up the evening sky just before the sun goes down.

Hsiao-Pi's mother had some difficulties speaking Mandarin. Not that she had a strong accent or pronounced words incorrectly; on the contrary, she had a very distinct articulation. But there were two things that gave her trouble: First, her Mandarin sentences were translations from the Taiwanese, which explained why she talked more slowly than other people; second, she talked very little, and it was almost as if she were gradually losing her ability to speak. Mr. and Mrs. Pi hardly talked to each other directly. They communicated via their children, often telling them things that were really meant for their spouse's ear. Mrs. Pi spoke Taiwanese with the children, and after a while, Mr. Pi somehow could understand what she was saying. One day, for example, Mrs. Pi would say to the kids in Taiwanese: "There are such big holes in your shoes; at New Year we'll have to buy new pairs for you!" On the following Sunday, Mr. Pi would take the kids into town and pick out new shoes for them at the Sheng-Sheng Shoe Store. Hsiao-Pi never came with them, but Mr. Pi always remembered to buy a pair for him, too. Usually he chose the right size, and if he didn't, he would go back to the store after work and get a pair that fit.

I remember one year's Mid-Autumn Festival when we went up to the T'e-Kuang Temple in the hills near our neighborhood to admire the full moon. On our way there, Uncle Pi was acting like a clown to entertain me and my sisters. He was very fond of kids, especially little girls, and sure enough he succeeded in making us shake with laughter. He even let our youngest sister ride on his shoulders, swaying to the left and the right like a dancing lion at a Chinese New Year festivity as he carried her all the way up the hill. He looked rather like a living God of Fortune, short and heavy. His head was especially prone to perspire profusely. Mrs. Pi took a cool towel out of a plastic bag and handed it to Uncle Pi, who wiped off the sweat, and then folded the towel neatly to put it back into the bag again. Later we sat in a pavilion and ate moon cakes and pomelos, the proper food for the occasion, while listening to Uncle Pi and our father recalling what the Mid-Autumn Festival was like on the mainland. Mrs. Pi ate little and talked even less, concentrating on the task of peeling pomelos and handing out segments to everybody. Otherwise she would use a goose feather fan to drive away the mosquitoes that were hovering about everybody's feet. Hsiao-Pi was running around, playing in front of the temple or at its back. Once in a while he came over to eat some pomelos, only to dash off again as soon as he was finished. He would never play with us girls, avoiding us at all times—unless he was playing pranks on us. The moon that night seemed to be particularly bright and round, and the steps of the pavilion were flooded with moonlight.

Every day at noon Mrs. Pi would come to school to bring Hsiao-Pi his lunchbox. In summer, a bottle of water would go with it to replace the one Hsiao-Pi had already emptied during the morning. When it was raining, even drizzling, she always brought him his raincoat. On cool days, she came to bring him his jacket—I don't remember any other mother who did so much for her kid. Like most boys, Hsiao-Pi hated to wear a raincoat or even to put on an extra piece of clothing when the weather was changing. And yet, though Hsiao-Pi was quite an obstinate little fellow, his mother—and only she—never needed to use harsh words or stern looks when dealing with him. He would obey her. Oh yes, he put on his jacket all right, but not without making a few adjustments to suit him. He would tie the sleeves into a knot in front of his neck, thus creating a little cloak. Even so, he had done what his mother had asked and put it on. And when it came to his raincoat, he would simply fit it loosely over his shoulders and fasten only the top button. When he was running in this outfit, he produced a delightful swooshing sound, probably imagining he was some kind of Zorro.

In junior high school, Hsiao-Pi was put in a class with a number of bad students. There, learning to smoke and fight, he mixed with bad boys and continually got into trouble. Every two or three days Uncle Pi would go to see Hsiao-Pi's teachers and try to hush things up, but Hsiao-Pi's misdeeds would still be announced on the school's bulletin board. As far as I was concerned, though, Hsiao-Pi was not a bad kid. One day on my way home from school, three boys barred my way on a lane by the Liu's home next to the food market. One of them announced my name, while another one said in a mean voice, "Now why does our little miss always act so proud?" I was quite baffled, for I didn't even know these young ruffians. The guy with the mean voice kept talking to me, "You think 'cause you're a model student, you're something better than the rest of us, don't ya? God, how phoney can you get?" Then he suddenly grabbed me by my hair and started to pull at it.

Exactly at that moment I heard Hsiao-Pi's voice coming from behind us, shouting at the boys, "Don't you guys touch her! She's my daddy's goddaughter!" I didn't know how those boys disappeared, I just heard Hsiao-Pi's voice saying, "Don't worry. Nobody's gonna bother you in the future."

At that time I was too flustered to say much, and when I tried to thank Hsiao-Pi later on, he would always avoid the topic, acting as if the whole thing had never happened. Several times when I was delivering the class register at the office, I would see Hsiao-Pi standing in the dean's office, the dean of students madly flailing his arms and yelling at Hsiao-Pi. Not that penalties and shouted lectures had any effect on Hsiao-Pi, since he himself never thought he had done anything wrong. Witnessing scenes like that, I usually felt chagrined, wishing very much that Hsiao-Pi was aware that I did not share other people's negative opinions of him.

In his third year at junior high, Hsiao-Pi stole money from Uncle Pi and spent it with some good-for-nothing friends. That money had been specially put aside by Uncle Pi to pay for the children's tuition. That night, everywhere in our house, we could hear the hollering voice of Uncle Pi as he cross-examined Hsiao-Pi next door. During the whole interrogation, Hsiao-Pi uttered not a single word. In his fury, Uncle Pi thrashed Hsiao-Pi with a leather hose. Halfway through the spanking, we could hear Hsiao-Pi screaming, "How can you hit me! You're not even my father!" Smack, smack—that was the sound of Mrs. Pi slapping Hsiao-Pi's face. And then silence began to settle on the house.

Uncle Pi fell heavily into his rattan chair. I'm absolutely sure that half our village was listening to what was going on in the Pi's place. The wind was soughing in the pines on the mountain nearby, and the old magazines lying forgotten in the yard made a rustling sound. After a long, long while, when everybody was beginning to think the show was over, Mrs. Pi's voice could suddenly be heard. She was obviously trying to make Hsiao-Pi kneel as punishment, but Hsiao-Pi resisted, and, gasping with rage, she shouted, "Get down on your knees, you ungrateful piece of shit! Who taught you to behave like this? I don't have a son like you. You ungrateful piece of dirt! He's not your father? Without him, where would you be now?" His voice also trembling with rage, Uncle Pi said, "I'm not your father. I don't deserve that you get on your knees before me, ha! Go find your father and kneel before him, then!"

Then it finally did become quiet. The heavy silence was only interrupted by occasional sobs and the distant sounds of weeping. Those were faintly audible each time I suddenly woke up from my light sleep that night.

On the very next morning, Mrs. Pi committed suicide by turning on the gas in the kitchen. When the kids came home from school in the afternoon, nobody came to open the door for them, so they decided to play with kids from the neighborhood. Later, when Mr. Pi came home from work by bus, he immediately felt something amiss. All help came too late; Mrs. Pi was already dead. She had left behind a kind of farewell letter using the few Chinese characters she knew: "To Chu-chia's father: I'm gone. To A-Chu: My boy, remember that I want you to be an obedient son to your father, or I won't find any peace in my grave! Chu-chia's mother, Fang-ying."

The people of our village set up a funeral committee. On the day of the burial, all of Uncle Pi's old friends from Henan Province showed up to take part in the procession. Hsiao-Pi and his two younger brothers knelt on one side of the mourning tent, kowtowing to all the mourners that came to pay their respects in front of Mrs. Pi's coffin. Hsiao-Pi in his hemp mourning garment seemed even skinnier and darker than usual. His huge mourning hat, too big for his head, fell over his face whenever he bent over to kowtow to the other mourners. At that time, I didn't really understand what had happened and why Mrs. Pi had killed herself, but the sight of the big mourning hat covering all of Hsiao-Pi's face was enough to make me cry.

Uncle Pi acted very calm and composed throughout the whole funeral, but when everything was over and he was sitting with my father to discuss some minor details that had still to be dealt with, the conversation made him break down in tears over Mrs. Pi's silliness. He went on and on about how he had never said a harsh word in ten years of marriage, and how he couldn't understand why Mrs. Pi had taken so seriously a few words that had obviously been spoken in a fit of rage. Yes, his wife had been much younger than he, could have been his daughter. He had been more than willing to provide her the things that were in his power to give: a stable home and loving care for the rest of her life. Hadn't she mocked his good intentions by committing suicide like that? Uncle Pi cried until he was weak with exhaustion. Then he talked about the arrangements that he made for Mrs. Pi's grave, mentioning details like its size and the material to be used for the gravestone. Everything had been meticulously planned. Uncle Pi sighed deeply and said, "This is all that I can do now. What else can I do?"

Hsiao-Pi decided to take the entrance examination for military school. Uncle Pi flew into a rage when he heard of it and insisted that Hsiao-Pi take the senior high school entrance exam instead. Hsiao-Pi defended his decision and explained that, first of all, he would never pass the senior high exam. Uncle Pi retorted, "In that case, you go to cram school for one year and try again." Hsiao-Pi went on that, second, military school had the big advantage of not charging any tuition. Now that made Uncle Pi so angry that he dragged Hsiao-Pi to his mother's memorial tablet and shouted, "Don't talk to me about tuition fees, young man! Your mother wanted you to get a good education, finish senior high, and go to college so that you may easily find a job and lead a decent life. So don't disappoint your mother and do as I say!" That wasn't the end of the argument, for Hsiao-Pi said that, third, after graduating from the military senior high he could directly enter a military academy without having to take any entrance exam. And military academy, Hsiao-Pi added, was every bit as good as college. Uncle Pi was trembling with rage as he roared, "Well, that's completely new to me, as good as college!" There was one thing that Hsiao-Pi had not mentioned during their argument, and that was that he wanted to make a clean break with the past. After all, he was still young, the future was wide open, and he wanted to start all over again.

In the end it was Hsiao-Pi's advisor, the dean of students, and the principal who united in their efforts to speak on Hsiao-Pi's behalf and eventually convinced Uncle Pi to let the boy have his way. On the day of Hsiao-Pi's graduation, one of the seats of honor was reserved for Uncle Pi to watch the ceremony. There he sat very erect, from beginning to end, his back straight and his two large hands placed firmly on his knees. Hsiao-Pi and one other boy had been recommended for admission to military senior high, and the two of them went up to the podium and were seen off with much praise and applause. Hsiao-Pi was wearing a red congratulatory sash across his breast that was knotted into a ball around his shoulder. Who do you think, Hsiao-Pi, was cheering the loudest and longest among all the audience?

The year after that, Uncle Pi retired from military service. He then left our village and moved elsewhere using his retirement annuity to open a grocery store together with his old friends from Henan Province. That was also the time when our whole village had to make space for modern apartment blocks that were part of a housing project. With houses to be pulled down soon, everybody was looking for a temporary home in the surrounding area. Uncle Pi also came back to handle the handing over of his old house. He brought some preserved food from his store for us kids, still calling us his "goddaughters." Before he left, he stood lost in thought in our yard, looking across the bamboo fence at his own house with its wilted roses and creeping oxalis.

I think that for Mrs. Pi, Uncle Pi was the only man she had ever had any deep feelings for. It seems that every love in this world is tainted in some way or other. And yet, she wanted so much for their relationship to work out so well that in the end, one flaw was enough to make death seem more attractive than life. Was that really Mrs. Pi's only choice?

The next time I saw Hsiao-Pi was during a junior high school class reunion that took place in a Western-style restaurant. On that occasion, somebody suddenly tapped me on the shoulder, and when I turned around, it was Hsiao-Pi! "Hsiao-Pi!" Everyone always called him by this nickname, and yet this was the first time that I had used it. In those long years since we had last seen each other, the skinny boy had turned into a handsome man, his dark tan indicating that he was bursting with health. Under his black eyebrows and eyelashes, his eyes were reminiscent of a rice paddy with the sprouts swaying gently in the wind; at times you can see the shimmering green reflections on the water below, but immediately they quiver again, leaving the water's surface dark once more. Yes, that was Hsiao-Pi, or first lieutenant of the ROC Air Force, Pi Chu-chia.

I asked him how Uncle Pi was. Hsiao-Pi laughed in a loud, clear voice, tipped his forehead with index finger and said, "You know, as my father's humble counselor in any situation, I came up with some ideas..." Then I learned that he had convinced Uncle Pi to expand his business. With

Hsiao-Pi's help and encouragement, Uncle Pi's store had been turned into a very modern grocery store, an undertaking that also received some support from the government. They had hired several employees to run the business and work as shop assistants, and Uncle Pi was very happy to find himself the big boss. In his leisure time, Uncle Pi would go and see his old friends from Henan, and they would drink tea and chat together or watch a Henan opera performance. Hsiao-Pi's two younger brothers both went to senior high school.

I was touched by his narration, and tears welled up in my eyes. I once more tried to thank him for coming to my rescue once when we both were still little kids. Hsiao-Pi listened with his head tilted to one side, sounding somewhat surprised as he said, "Oh, really?" I continued to tell him how I remembered one time when he was being punished and yelled at by the dean of students. Amazed and amused, he said again, "Oh, really?"

That was when I decided to write down the story of Hsiao-Pi.

* From Chu T'ien-wen's *Hua-yi chien-sheng* 《花憶前生》 (*A Flower Remembers Her Previous Lives*) (Taipei: Rye Field Publishing Co., 1996). Originally published in *Hsaio-pi-te ku-shih* 《小畢的 故事》 (*The Story of Hsiao-Pi*) (Taipei: San San Bookstore, 1983).

CHAPTER 3

THE PARTY GIRL

酒會的女人

Lin Tai-man 林黛嫚

(Translated by David van der Peet 范德培)

In telling this story, it is certainly not my intention to reveal any secrets from other people's lives. I simply have to vent my sheer shock and astonishment. It wasn't just that this woman had the same dreams and ideas I did. What really got to me was this: While I was just thinking about all those things, making big plans that were elaborate and absolutely flawless in my imagination, she actually went out and made it happen.

On the day I met her, we somehow got into conversation at one of those high-class social events. Only later did I realize that, after checking out the party for a bit, she had deliberately chosen me to tell her story to—or should I say, to impress me with it.

That day, I had made my entry as usual. The host and hostess were standing at the entrance welcoming the guests. With countless media cameras leveled at that spot, constantly going click, click, click for fear of missing the arrival of a major bigwig, I managed to slip inside unnoticed behind a legislator and his surrounding entourage of assistants. The truth was, I might as well have walked right up to the hosts, shaken their hands, and said something like "Congratulations!" or "How're you doing?" because the question "Do I know this person?" would never even have crossed their minds. But even after attending such events so many times, I could never drum up the courage to give it a try.

Having entered, I quickly found a large pillar to lean against, and as a waiter walked past I nimbly snatched a glass of champagne from his tray. It was a pity I'd never been able to drink a lot—my personal record at one of those dinner parties was two glasses of white wine and three of champagne, drunk over the course of the entire event. If I could really hold my liquor, I'd get a chance to finish a bottle or two of really expensive, high-end hooch at every go, for free!

I had picked a good spot. To my left and right were VIPs and dignitaries, all dressed up for the occasion. As I raised my eyes to the ceiling, they were dazzled by the reflections of the luxurious ballroom's splendid interior. Directly in the middle of the central buffet table rose a thick column of ice into the speckled disco lighting that illuminated the fresh flowers and exquisite delicacies below. Since I didn't want to draw other people's attention by monopolizing my spot, I moved away from the pillar after twenty minutes and strolled over to the one on the opposite side of the hall. I lingered there for another twenty minutes before scuttling back to my original vantage point.

I was very familiar with this particular hotel. In Taipei, no other place was more famous for its cocktail parties and dinner receptions, and so it was also the one I'd been to most frequently. I felt that this should be the ideal place for the plan I had in my head to succeed.

That morning, I hadn't drunk any milk. I didn't actually like milk, but I forced myself to drink a glass or two every day to balance my calcium intake and to make up for the two daily cups of coffee I also consumed. The thing was, though, that lately I'd felt that I was getting a bit plump around the waist, and I blamed it on the coffee and milk. But since there was no way I'd be able to quit the coffee—you need some things to spice up your life—I had to sacrifice health and nutrition instead. Consequently, I'd had just a glass of water before the reception, and after two rather quickly downed glasses of white wine on what was basically an empty stomach, I could already feel the alcohol circulating through every part of my system.

The lights began to look just a tiny bit blurry and I had reached about the right degree of tipsiness, finally feeling brave enough to go and talk to people. I was just about to look for someone to exchange a bit of small talk with when a person materialized right in front of me, looking at me.

"You're here alone? Not easy to find someone you know with the place so packed with people. Just now, I was sure I'd recognized someone I know standing over there talking to someone, but when I wanted to go over and say hi, he had already disappeared, just like that."

She was about half a head taller than me, so if I didn't lift my head my eyes were at the same level as the slightly curled corners of her cherry mouth. Standing this close to her, I couldn't get a good look at the woman. I stepped back a little so that my back came to rest against the cool marble pillar behind me. Now I could give her a good once-over, and I noticed that her stomach was flat to the point of almost being concave. She wore a charcoal satin dress with delicate straps that revealed much of her back. Her shoulders and gaunt collarbone caught the eye and contributed to the overall impression of a fragile yet sexy skinniness. The faint goosebumps on her skin, a result of the very cold air-conditioning, made her look even more attractive.

My description isn't that bad, is it? After all, I've been messing around at various second-rate tabloid magazines for several years, not-too-classy publications with titles like *Inside Report, Exposed,* or *Eye-Witness News.* Even as a minor editor, I've had ample opportunity to read through the nonsense "reports" and "interviews" concocted by so-called journalists, and have naturally picked up some of the vocabulary usually employed in accounts and portrayals of the upper class, of stars, and other famous people.

I hadn't even got a good look at her face yet, but already I knew that she was a real looker. And indeed, as our eyes met, I was immediately touched by the limpid beauty of large eyes that were sparkling with energy. The truth was, I had never been this close to a person this beautiful. Like a movie star, she was. Of course, even the kind of low-grade gutter press I was working for had to cultivate some direct contacts with top idols and superstars, but none of that happened at the level of an inconsequential editor.

She gave an attractive smile as she carelessly fingered the pearl earrings peeping through her bobbed hair, "Hey, you got a really horny look on your face, you know that?"

That remark made me go completely red in the face. There I was, a rather shy person used to hiding in corners and observing people from a safe distance, to scrutinizing all those ladies and gentlemen to my heart's content, and I had completely forgotten that this person was standing right in front of me and talking to me. Very slowly, almost stuttering, I squeezed out an "I'm sorry" in a voice that was so thin and weak as to be almost inaudible.

But she shrugged it all off with a "Don't worry, I'm used to it."

"To be honest, I hardly know anybody in here, either. So would you mind chatting with me for a little?"

There was nothing I would've liked more, of course. It's more than awkward to be at one of these events and have absolutely no one to talk to. When that happens, you start walking about the room uncomfortably in an effort to avoid the attention of the roaming eyes of those who seem to be casually chatting. That's also why everybody's always holding a drink in their hands: sipping at your glass now and then gives you an occupied air.

"My name's Hsu Tsui-hsuan. What's yours?"

"Chang Tzu-ju," I made up a name off the top of my head. Who knew if Hsu Tsui-hsuan was her real name!

She laughed in a somewhat odd manner, as if she knew exactly what I was thinking. Or maybe it was me being too suspicious; maybe she was just trying to be friendly. After all, I always seem to give people the impression of being extremely nervous and uptight. That's what all my colleagues at the magazine say, anyway.

"You see that guy over there by the ice sculpture, the one with the red hair? His entire outfit is Armani, including those shoes. God I love those shoes, elegant and stylish, but still very soft and comfortable. I have to say, though, he really should dye his hair another color. Guys with red hair are such wussies. Nothing but talk, they are."

"And that other dude, who's talking to the stunning Ms. Lin, he's the boss of some movie company. Got more women than sons, he has. Not the smartest cookie in the box. When he kicks the bucket one day, those women will come after his sons like sharks in the water. They'll milk them for all they can get..."

"The one in the yellow suit, with the earring, he's so obviously gay. And still he goes and marries a woman—all façade. I mean, look at him, that garish yellow suit is just screaming, 'Fellas, come and get me!'"

Hsu Tsui-hsuan had a very pleasant, cultivated voice and spoke Mandarin without the slightest accent, which made her sound like a top-notch broadcaster. The most amazing thing was the pitch of her voice: not too high, not too low, very flat and smooth, and not betraying any emotion at all. Even though she was gossiping and saying nasty things about people, you'd never have guessed as much from her cool, composed demeanor. So it was that whenever people walked past us and accidentally caught a phrase or two, it never quite grabbed their attention.

Everything she said surprised and astonished me. How did she know so much? Where did she get those penetrating insights from? In my amazement, I had already finished the glass of white wine in my hand, and before I knew it, another one.

"Hey, you shouldn't drink any more, or you'll make a fool of yourself."

But it was already too late, it seemed. My cheeks felt vaguely numb, and my mouth was moving of its own accord; I could hear myself giggling foolishly.

"Dear me," she sighed and grabbed me under the armpits. Applying mild force, she half-dragged and half-led me out of the ballroom.

I was just a bit tiddly, not really drunk. That is, although I wasn't quite in control of all my movements anymore, my mind was still perfectly clear and alert. Still, I didn't put up much resistance, since I didn't want to stay anyway. Hsu Tsui-hsuan was so much more interesting than any of the other people at that reception, and wherever she was going, I couldn't wait to go with her and learn something.

She waved down a taxi. "I don't live that far from here, but I'd be exhausted if I had to drag you all the way there on foot in this warm weather." She gave the driver an address on one of the small alleys off Chung-shan North Road.

After a ride through tortuous lanes and labyrinthine alleys, the cab came to a halt in front of an old-fashioned apartment block. As we got out of the car, she paid the fifty-dollar fare with a one-hundred-dollar bill and told the driver to keep the change. Before I even had a chance to ask why she tipped the man so generously, she explained that one should always be nice to those who have to do physical labor to make a living, adding that precisely because she wasn't one of them, she understood how hard that was. "Also," she went on, "what's a hundred dollars when you just drank so much white wine for free, eh?"

The place must have been in one of the old districts established by the Japanese, not that I would ever get a good grasp of Taipei's layout with its convoluted streets and alleys. One time, I happened to be near the Kuang-hua Mall when I decided to try a shortcut and turned onto a small lane, confident that after a few twists and turns I should come out where I wanted to. Turned out I was wrong. After about half an hour, I had completely lost any sense of direction, but in my stubbornness I refused to give up. I told myself there had to be some kind of system to the way all these alleys and lanes were arranged and connected. So I kept walking, with dogged determination, for a full three hours before I finally capitulated, standing by the roadside, defeated and tired, a picture of utter misery.

Although the building was old, it did have an elevator, a clear indication that at some point this must have been a rather posh place. Hsu Tsui-hsuan pressed the button for the top floor. By now, I no longer had to lean on her. She looked at me and said, "You've pretty much sobered up, haven't you?" In reply I laughed again, only this time it wasn't a drunk giggle, but more of an embarrassed titter. Now that my tipsiness was gone, so was my Dutch courage, it seemed. I was back to being the usual me, the person who didn't dare to make a move at a reception before she began to feel the effects of her first drink.

I stepped out of the elevator to find three apartments close by. But Hsu Tsui-hsuan went past them, and up a flight of stairs. That's right, single women in Taipei usually have no other choice but to rent a pad in illegal structures built on top of tenement buildings. It was the same for me; mine was on Chi-lin Road.

As soon as Hsu Tsui-hsuan had opened the door to her room, we were hit by a wave of hot air. As if it weren't sultry enough outside, inside the air was positively suffocating. There wasn't a single window, and the door was the only opening through which air could escape or enter. Her room was adjoined by more illegal lodgings to the left and right. Good thing that I was hardened to this kind of environment. Believe it or not,

I had lived in even worse dumps than that. Once I rented a basement room, reached by dark stairs and separated from many other mutually adjoining ones by thin wooden planks so that not the slightest bit of space was wasted. Every room was furnished with just a bed, a desk, and a plastic wardrobe. And, mind you, often you had to share one of these tiny rooms with someone else. This was the only kind of place I could afford when I'd just come to Taipei.

Hsu Tsui-hsuan switched on the fan and turned it up to full speed, but at first even the wind was hot. After a while we got used to it, though. When she felt that I had adjusted to the temperature in the room, she closed the door, since it was facing the toilet.

"What would you like to drink? Coke or oolong tea?" A small fridge stood in one corner of the room. She went and opened it, bending from the waist while keeping her knees straight, a posture that allowed me to fully appraise her amazing figure. Ah, what perfect proportions! When I didn't say anything in reply to her question, she simply handed me a can of Diet Coke. "Don't worry, it's low-cal."

She opened another can for herself, took a sip, and put it down on a table next to her. Then she proceeded to change in front of me. It was only when she took off the dress that I noticed she wasn't wearing a bra, only two tiny adhesive nipple covers. After she had put on her pajamas, she reached inside the loose top and took those off as well.

"Expensive clothes require a lot of care, and that costs money. That's why I always get changed first thing after coming home. And I don't wear bras because they would ruin the effect of the body-hugging dresses I wear. You see, this kind of light and smooth fabric just won't look good with the contours of a bra showing through it. Not neat. And when guys put their hands on your back and discover that you're not wearing a bra, they'll start fantasizing. You've practically won them over already." Hsu Tsui-hsuan was standing akimbo in front of her dressing mirror, hands resting on her slender waist, as she continued, "The one thing women can't afford to be is fat. When you're fat, you'll look grubby, dumb, and clumsy—a slattern. But it's hard work to maintain a slim figure. For me it's easy because I have an ulcer. No matter how much I eat, I just don't gain any weight. But you, you really should pay more attention to your diet."

Now she'd made me flush again. I knew perfectly well that I needed to pay more attention to my diet! But I just loved to eat, simply couldn't resist the temptation of food. Junk food in particular was irresistible: cakes, chocolates, hamburgers, Coke, all the things that we could rarely or never afford when I was a child. But even as I was flushing, I was also feeling somewhat confused. Wasn't this woman strange, bringing a woman back home she knew absolutely nothing about, just like that, and then inexplicably talking to her about all sorts of things? Then again, wasn't my behavior just as weird? Following her home just like that, and listening to her outpourings, watching her move about. While all these bewildered thoughts were still tumbling through my mind, she had already sat down next to me on the bed.

"What did you say your name was again?"

"Chang Chih-ju." That's what I had told her earlier, wasn't it?

She laughed again, let out a sigh, and lighted herself a Virginia Slim. "Looks like I've got a lot to teach you."

"Teach me?" What was that supposed to mean? I didn't ask the second question out loud. I knew she'd go on talking, anyway.

She let out a puff of smoke. "I'm leaving here tomorrow. I'm finally putting all this behind me. God, I'm so tired."

"It'll take a while to tell my whole story. I'll go into a lot of detail, you know, and tell it slowly. But you don't have anything better to do at the moment anyway, am I right? So, I'll just talk and you listen. Please don't interrupt me, or I'll lose the thread of what I'm saying. If you have any questions, please wait until I'm finished. When I first saw you at that reception today, I figured you were the same kind of person I am. So I think my personal experiences might be useful to you. Should I be mistaken about this, and you're after all a different person from me, it doesn't matter, either. Just listen to it as you'd listen to a story, 'cause it's an interesting story that I've got to tell.

"My real name is not Hsu Tsui-hsuan, just like yours isn't Chang Tzu-ju or Chang Chih-ju or whatever. It doesn't really matter, of course, it's just a name. Deep down inside, parents don't really believe that if they call their child 'Mei-li' it will actually grow up to be beautiful; or if they name it 'Tsung-ming' it will turn out to be particularly intelligent. Otherwise, all children would have auspicious names like 'Hao-ming' or 'Fu-kui'—who doesn't want an easy life or wealth and position for their offspring? Basically, those parents who ask a fortune-teller to carefully pick a good name according to astrological principles, and pay attention to the number and order of strokes in the characters of the name—well, those are usually the parents who are able to provide their children with a very decent standard of living. Parents who are too busy eking out a living, on the other hand, naturally won't have the time and energy to bother with such niceties like choosing a special name for their kids."

Wow, just like she had said, she was quite the talker! Lots of detail, indeed. Unfortunately, I was a rather fidgety kind of person. From early childhood, sitting still for prolonged periods of time had never been my thing; otherwise I'd have been a much better student and might have gotten much better grades. And then my life might be looking very different. But there wasn't any use in wasting much thought on these things. They were in the past, and I was here, in the present. I wasn't one to dwell much on the past, but Hsu Tsui-hsuan didn't seem to mind doing exactly that and appeared determined to start at the very beginning. Fortunately, it wasn't as if there wasn't anything to distract me a bit. As I sat there, sipping at my nice, cool Diet Coke, I took a closer look at Hsu Tsui-hsuan's wardrobe. When she'd hung up her dress earlier, she hadn't pulled up the zipper of the plastic closet. She obviously wanted me to get a good look at it, so that I might get an idea of what kind of outfits I needed to add to my wardrobe. She didn't have a lot of clothes, but each piece was neatly hung up and separated according to the seasons. Most of them were designer suit dresses of a similar cut, but there were also one-piece dresses, knee-length skirts, and little coats, all in pastel colors and designed to give people exactly the impression that I'd had when I'd seen her at the cocktail party that day: decorous and elegant, yet not without a subtle spark of youthful vigor. A well-bred young woman who yet wouldn't disappoint you in bed—wasn't that exactly the type that men were looking for in their future wives?

"I've always wanted to succeed, right from the start, when I was just a little girl. But these days, everybody wants to make it big, so there's nothing special about that, and there is no need for a reason whatsoever. If people didn't have this compelling urge to climb the ladder of success and recognition, there wouldn't be all those scientists and inventors who come up with so many ways and things to make our lives easier and better. But of course there are many forms of success, and many ways to it. Like that young female city councilor who inherited her father's political capital when she was only twenty-three and became a renowned politician herself. Me, I don't have that kind of background. Neither do I have the necessary talent or skills to make a lot of money and retire a filthy rich entrepreneur by the time I'm forty or fifty, or maybe sixty. And in terms of looks—you may well think that I'm not bad-looking at all. But the truth is, while I'm certainly not unattractive, I'm hardly movie-star material, either. Far from it! And to really make it in the showbiz industry, it takes more than just a great body, beautiful looks, or even outstanding social skills. The most important thing is luck, getting that one break you need. And that's something I can't control.

"So, what kind of success is it then that I'm after? First of all, I want lots of money. It doesn't have to be the kind of money that the Tsais or the Wus have, but enough to allow me to pamper myself, and to allow my family to do the same. I don't want my parents to be hawking vegetables on the streets for the rest of their lives. Or at least, I want them to have their own stall at a decent supermarket. And I don't want my younger brothers and sisters to have to work their way through college like I did. I don't want them to have to live in this kind of hole with wooden partitions. I want them to get a good shot at success themselves, want them to be able to study and go abroad without having to worry about where the money's coming from.

"Next, I want to enjoy a life of elegance and taste. I wouldn't wanna marry someone like Mr. 'The Road Is Mine' Liu who owns practically the entire Chung-shan North Road. The first thing he did after getting himself a wife was to fire his accountant. Now all his wife does is sit at home all day keeping the books. Not for me, that. The best would be to live abroad, in a high-class residential area in a rich, advanced country. Or maybe a developing country, and then I'd have a nurse for each of my children. I'd travel around the world, going to Paris to watch some opera, to New York to see some plays on Broadway, and to Japan to see Mount Fuji...

"Now don't you laugh at me. I know I'm just dreaming, but it's better to have dreams like this than to have no ambitions at all. I certainly don't plan to spend my entire life mired in mediocrity. There was this elderly woman, a fishmonger. She and my mother were always selling their wares together on the streets. From when I was very little, she was forever going on about how she wanted me to become her son's wife, as if it was the most natural and logical thing in the world that a veggie monger's daughter should marry a fishmonger's son. I hated that. Now, since I can't realize my dreams by myself, the only way to do it is by marrying a rich man."

Hsu Tsui-hsuan was speaking in a serious tone, and her voice was resonant with conviction. Her white face was now flushed with a kind of indignant agitation, her bright eyes shining with a focused concentration, as if that dream of hers was floating right in front of her eyes, like a balloon floating tantalizingly within her reach. All she had to do was stretch out her arms and grab it, hold on to it tight, and it would be hers forever.

During Hsu Tsui-hsuan's lengthy prologue, I had let my eyes roam over the whole room. The double bed I was sitting on took up pretty much half of the available space. To its right stood a small desk that served as a dressing table, and to its left was a low wooden table with a TV on it (no idea if it worked). On the bedhead cabinet were strewn a CD Walkman connected to two small speakers and several CDs. Next to the door was the closet, and next to that the little fridge. It took only about five minutes to take it all in. All the bare necessities, but little more. I sighed inwardly, thinking how many young women in this bright and bustling metropolis were living in this kind of quarters, spending their days and nights dreaming of the big break.

"My room's pretty basic, right? Everything in here has a specific purpose. Like those magazines on the bedhead cabinet, they're all the latest issues of Vogue. Can't afford to read older issues, because every day counts when it comes to staying ahead of fashion. Those magazines are my most important source of the latest info on famous brands, the male psychology, and what's happening in the world at large.

"And don't think it can't be done: I'm almost there," she went on.

"There was no way I'd go to a normal senior high school, even though my grades were good enough—I could've had my pick of the best schools. But think about it: going to senior high school, you have to study all the time. You are lucky if you don't end up severely shortsighted, and you certainly don't have time to stay in good shape and maintain a good figure. And besides, studying useless stuff like physics, chemistry, math, or the Three Principles of the People is just a major waste of time. And after three years of that, there's still no guarantee that you'll be able to pass the university entrance exam. So what I did was to pick some junior college, didn't really matter what kind. The whole point was to gain access to university through a side door. Do you have any idea how easy it is to transfer from junior college to a private university's night school program? The geography department was looking for thirty-some transfer students every year, and although I only scored a little more than a hundred points in the entrance test, and just three points in the subject General Geography, I was still accepted. I messed about for a year, and then I switched to the French department. It meant an extra year, since I had to start as a freshman again, but that didn't matter. I was working in the daytime, anyway, making money."

Hearing this, I had to sigh again. If only I had met Hsu Tsui-hsuan a few years earlier, I could've saved myself the trouble and pain of going through the hell that is the university entrance examination. I still remember how I performed well above my usual level in the senior high school entrance exam, getting a better score than during all my three years of junior high, allowing me to claim my first preference school with a total score a half-point above the threshold. My parents were on cloud nine. But of course the fact remained that I had over-performed on that exam, and in the end I had to repeat the first year in senior high. Later, I failed to get into university at my first attempt. The following year, I managed to gain admission into the night school Chinese department of Providence University, largely on account of being a girl. It was the only school I could get into with my 202 points in the entrance exam, but as a boy, I would still have needed ten more points to qualify even for the last-option university, Feng Chia. And so I was stuck in the sticks of Shalu for the next five years. Apart from poring over weighty tomes and—at least—picking up some professional skills that came in handy working as an editor, I came away with nothing from my time there.

"During my time as a student, I also dated young men. As you can see, I'm not exactly an ugly duckling, and so I had quite a few boyfriends, some of which I got along with rather well. But you have to understand that those who were in it for the same reasons as me wouldn't be interested in me—naturally, they wanted a young lady from a rich family, the fast lane to wealth and an easy life and all that. And then there are those honest types who have to work their way up slowly, step by step, through hard work and diligence. But that's not for me, I wouldn't have the patience to wait for that. In the beginning, I would even fall in love, you know, but then I discovered that love is a very uneconomical thing. It costs money and it costs time, not to mention all the emotions you have to invest in it. And when you break up, it breaks your heart and harms your health. In the end, I just didn't have the energy for it anymore. Unless it was someone who looked like he might make it big, I wouldn't even bother to deal with him.

"It's a long, drawn-out process, looking for the right guy like that, and it's neither easy nor fun. It's like doing business or investing in the stock market. There's always the risk of failure. I know this from firsthand experience. After entering university, I started to go to all the balls and parties thrown by every department. Of ten dances, nine would be solely for the purpose of investigating my dance partner's family background, but I'd reward myself for all the hard work with one jitterbug that I did just for the enjoyment of it. And I wasn't just digging for the lowdown on my respective dance partners, I'd also pump them for information about other potential prospects. Eventually, I set my eyes on a student from the economics department. His family owned half the buses in Taipei, as well as several department stores, and while they may not have been obscenely wealthy, I could see a lot of potential there. Another reason I liked him, apart from his very promising background, was that he had a little canine tooth that looked really cute and gave him a childlike, innocent air when he was laughing. Still looked very attractive, mind you. I wanted someone who I could easily control, and this guy appeared naive and trusting enough.

"I began to go after him, with determination and discretion. I found out his schedule and started to sit in on general education classes he was in. I created several 'chance meetings' to make sure he knew who I was before I made my first official move at one of the university balls. And sure enough, I had him chasing me after that. We started to date, just like normal university students, going to the movies, drinking black bubble tea, going bowling or singing at KTVs. I kept him dangling, going out with him for a few days and then keeping my distance for a few days.

I had decided that this was the fish I intended to catch, and so I wanted to make sure that he was hooked, and hooked good.

"After we had been going out for a little more than half a year, and had declared our love for each other, he took me to meet his family. And after that, after meeting his parents, the whole thing was suddenly over. Just like that. He stopped calling me, and of course I knew exactly what that meant. But I couldn't reconcile myself to it ending so abruptly, without even quite knowing why. So I went to see him, asking him to give me a reason, or at least come up with some excuse. He said, 'My father thinks you're too much for me to handle, and that I'm not the right guy for you. He also told me that once I get my doctorate, he'll find a nice young lady from a good family for me.' I was glad that he told me the plain truth instead of trying to feed me some lame excuses. I didn't blame him, honestly. Everybody has the right to make their choice, and to demand certain things.

"I often think of his innocent smile. I have long lost the ability to smile a genuine smile like that, so romantic and sincere." At this point, Hsu Tsui-hsuan crushed the empty Diet Coke can in her hand, stood up, and threw it in the wastebasket. Then she went to the fridge and got herself another can. As her head was turned toward me for one short moment, I thought I could see a single tear rolling from the corner of one eye, but it disappeared in an instant and was gone—irrevocably gone like the innocence of her smile.

She had noticed that I'd seen her tear. "After all this time, it still hurts to think about it. The tougher a woman appears on the outside, the more fragile she is emotionally. That's because it's damn hard work to maintain that cool exterior, and when you exhaust all your strength doing that, there aren't any defenses left to protect your heart. The slightest emotional turbulence can completely upset you. Well, that's just a bit of advice on the side; I don't mean to teach you how to read women. So let's get back to our main topic, how to chase men, or rather how to make them chase you.

"I had suffered defeat, but at least I had learned something from my failure. I realized that my past was a liability. I had done so much to improve myself, had learned English and French, swimming and dancing, and had learned to read time. Every penny of my hard-earned money I invested in acquiring the right skills and relevant knowledge. Only the piano and the violin I never learned, it was just too expensive. But I sang well, knew how to appreciate a good drop, I was pretty good at bowling and tennis, and I even knew a little bit about classical music and opera. But no matter how hard I tried, I couldn't substitute a glorious family background for my working class one. I would always be the daughter of a vegetable hawker. I wasn't even able to afford a decent place to live in. So I had to change my strategy.

"Fortunately I had not invested everything in the ill-fated affair with 'Little Mr. Future Transport Tycoon,' or 'Little Canine,' as I also called him. Otherwise, I would have lost my most powerful weapon. You can always fall in love again, but you can lose your virginity only once. And men place a lot of emphasis on this. The more successful they are, the more they care about it. Whether their future wife is a virgin is more important to them than whether or not she truly loves them.

"While on a rational level I could sympathize to some degree with Little Canine, and understand why he rejected me, on an emotional level it was much harder to forgive him. I was still hurting. I don't know when or under what circumstances you first started to go to cocktail parties. For me, success came right on the heels of my big disappointment.

"But first came graduation day. I was looking my very best, wearing my most fashionable outfit: a cream-yellow Chanel dress, proper and distinguished. I wore my hair tied in a knot, revealing the beautiful curve of my neck and shoulders. I also wore the most elegant makeup and carried an indigo Nina Ricci handbag. I took a taxi to Tianmu and paid a visit to Little Canine. His parents' home was actually in Sanchung, but he had a place of his own in Tianmu, one of his family's many pieces of real estate. After leaving his place, I jumped on a bus. It was almost empty, as it was around noontime. The strong aircon quickly dried my sweat and helped to cool my feelings of anger and indignation. I stared emptily out the bus window. Outside, the bustling scenes of Chung-shan North Road were drifting by, and as the bus was driving past Taipei's newest and most fancy hotel, I suddenly came to my senses. I was still here, and everything I wanted was still right in front of me, waiting for me to come and get it: money and power, wealth and status. My first attempt had failed—so what? Taipei was full of rich and powerful people; I couldn't afford to be depressed any longer, not for another minute. My strong fighting spirit was rekindled as I thought how befitting it was that graduation should mark the end of my learning days. Now it was time to put my experience and knowledge to good use. So I decided on the spot that I would walk right into that big fancy hotel, take a seat in the restaurant and treat myself to an expensive steak meal to invigorate and encourage myself.

"Before that day, Taipei's grand hotels hadn't exactly been my turf. I'd been to a few for a dinner party or just to stroll about aimlessly. This one, though, which counted international stars among its previous guests, I now entered for the first time. I had no idea which floor I'd have to go to for a steak, but I didn't want to ask anybody for directions. Why bother, I had more than enough time on my hands to explore the place slowly. So I kept walking further inside, and upstairs, always following the countless flower baskets along the route, until at last, following a group of smartly dressed ladies and gentlemen, I found myself at the entrance to the banquet hall. The host of an international cocktail party was in the process of welcoming the guests, shaking the hands of everyone entering the hall. When it was my turn, the host didn't hesitate the least bit to shake my hand with the same warm enthusiasm as that of everyone else. It was as if I were one of them, one of the distinguished guests. As I followed the crowd inside, I was immediately intimidated by the sheer magnificence and splendor of the sumptuous interior. You know what I'm talking about, because you've seen it all yourself, so I don't need to dwell on the details here. I found a corner where I could observe everyone and everything at my leisure, watching, listening, and thinking. Thanks to my good language skills I had no problems following the conversations around me. I could see it all very clearly now. In my mind's eye, everything was falling into place—I could discern the minutest details of my future as if I were looking at a realistic oil painting executed in the most vivid strokes and brightest colors. Finally my dreams were coming to fruition."

As Hsu Tsui-hsuan was talking about her first time at a cocktail party, I was reminiscing about mine. It had been a medium-sized cocktail party I'd gone to with the publisher of our magazine. I was immediately hooked, both by the overwhelming material delights and the fascinating human aspect of such occasions. I loved to watch people, especially members of high society. It was like confirming the reality of the luxurious and extravagant life I knew only from the many Hollywood movies I had watched. I also noticed that except for a few people who were really working the party, most of those present didn't know much more than a handful of the other guests. In fact, most of them only interacted with one or two other people. Some recognized exactly two names on the invitation card: the host's and their own. And I wouldn't have been surprised if there also were others like me who didn't even know the host. Everybody was there for one reason only, to meet other people who might further their interests. And there I was, enjoying myself in this place where human relations were a strange mix of intimate proximity and aloof distance.

Captivated by it all, I began to figure out ways to satisfy my addiction. The small number of invitations one received as a minor magazine editor was not enough for me, and so I started to secretly open the invitations of the publisher and of the senior CEO of our magazine. I'd memorize the time, address, and occasion of the event, but this method had the disadvantage that I often had to be very careful to avoid running into my superiors. Consequently, I began to scan the newspapers and listen to the radio for announcements of social events. I'd even go to the grand hotels in person to make roundabout inquiries and screen out the second-rate events. Then I'd dress to the nines, just like Hsu Tsui-hsuan, and mingle with the illustrious guests, pretending to be one of them. My objective was also the same as hers, to meet someone who would take care of me for the rest of my life. Of course, the difference between me and Hsu Tsui-hsuan was that I never had any deeper conversations with any of the strangers at those receptions. At most, I would make some meaningless small talk with one or two other young women who were just as alone and uneasy as myself. That was only logical, since I was much less well prepared than Hsu Tsui-hsuan had been. I seriously sucked at foreign languages, I didn't know enough about current events and famous brands, and I simply had no idea how to make the first move. I was just hanging around and waiting, waiting for some millionaire to walk right up to me in my corner and politely introduce himself.

"Success came within a year. Tomorrow, I'll be going to France together with a promising young French diplomat. To stay with his family and get married, that is. In one year, he'll be appointed to a post in South America. And in the future, since he has a Chinese wife, it's very possible that he'll be transferred back to Taiwan, or assigned to a post in Hong Kong, Beijing, or Shanghai."

Hsu Tsui-hsuan's sentences had been getting shorter and more succinct, and her voice had dropped almost to a whisper. She gave a long sigh. Tiredness was clearly showing in her face, even through the makeup she hadn't bothered to remove. She lay back with her limbs stretched out, and seemed to fall asleep almost at once. She was lying absolutely still now, even her eyelids weren't twitching anymore.

I guessed her last remarks had been the conclusion of her narrative. She hadn't given me an opportunity to ask any questions, but the truth was that I didn't really feel like asking her anything. She had already shown me the way, now it was up to me to make things happen. Seeing that she was apparently fast asleep, I decided to leave without disturbing her. I got up cautiously, hoping that the spring mattress wouldn't bounce too much. I just wanted to walk away quietly, disappear from Hsu Tsui-hsuan's life without leaving the slightest trace.

Before stepping out of the room, I took one last look at her. It was a long, hard look, because I knew I would never see her again, but I didn't want to forget what she looked like—my "life mentor."

While I was standing there, wondering whether it was already too late for me to follow in her footsteps, and hoping that I'd be able to take the same smooth shortcut to success, I suddenly heard her voice, thick with sleep, "Please close the door when you leave."

When I walked away, there was a new urgency in my steps. There was a lot I still had to do. Before I had entered that room, I had only been a leisurely observer at those cocktail parties. But from now on, I'd be a serious player.

* From Lin Tai-Man's 林黛嫚 *Lin Tai-Man tuan-pien Hsiao-shuo hsuan-chi*《林黛嫚短篇小說選集》(*The Collection of Short Stories of Lin Tai-Man*) (Taipei: The Commercial Press, 2006, 23–42).

Chapter 4

Taipei Train Station

台北車站

Tsai Su-fen 蔡素芬

(Translated by Daniel J. Bauer 鮑端磊)

It was a time when society's ability to indulge itself in consumer goods had expanded at a tremendous rate, when there wasn't even a hint of a slow-down in sight. Masses of people came pouring into the city. They rushed in from the suburbs by train or bus to go to work or school. This great mob of humanity clogged the streets and avenues, turning them into numerous wriggling, crawling worms. Buses dashed over streets, their metallic sides aglow in the light. The shine and swish they left in their wake enveloped the city as if with fish scales that flashed with every move.

Modern high-rises shot upward from gigantic graveyards where not a soul used to pass without holding their breath. Other skyscrapers, replete with glass frames, the handiwork of skilled workers and architects, towered among shabby old buildings. It was as if a great soaring peacock had outstretched its wings beneath the rays of a brilliant sun. In fine restaurants, delicate ladies and cultivated gentlemen enjoyed the riches of abalone, shark's fins, and other gourmet fare. All of this showed that the city had arrived. It had reached the pinnacle of modernity and luxury and comfort. Money unspent and left over could now go for decorations in buildings or exquisite culinary delights for people not the least bit hungry.

The Taipei train station bore the brunt of it all—this entire amalgam of people, vehicles, and roads—and was stuffed to the gills on delicacies so sumptuous they strained the station's heart and taxed its inner organs. It was so overstuffed that it made low wheezing sounds as it spoke. Every day people squeezed through the station into the city for work or school. Others changed buses, headed for their hometown, or rushed to the airport, stomping step by step on its very heartstrings in their hurry. Surrounding roads couldn't help but turn into slowly moving rivulets of blood that flowed laboriously, causing traffic to thicken and then to clot. A tide of people wasted countless time on the roads, driving, riding, or just waiting. How they wished for a few hours to be added to each day to compensate for the time they'd lost on the road, so they could meticulously execute the career plans they had hatched for years.

Six different platforms at the station meant several directions. A family with bags and suitcases of all sizes appeared at Platform One, having just flown down a staircase in near panic. At first the family had gone to the wrong platform. From there it scampered to Platform One, and boarded the train there. The husband, who was in charge of the large suitcase, stepped aboard on the heels of his wife at the very minute the train started to move. She had crammed herself into the front of the car, giving him a piece of her mind for his clumsiness in finding the right platform. He had made her heartbeat quicken by twenty percent. She was afraid their six-year-old boy would tumble to the tracks beneath the wheels, and held him so tightly she left purple marks on his little wrist. After the husband bent his head and studied the seat numbers on all four tickets, he put them back into his pocket. He patted the outside of the pocket for good measure, and felt their hard shape inside. The tickets lying safe and sound at the bottom of his pocket, he could relax now and lead his wife (she was still angry at him) and two sons through the congested aisle ahead to look for their seats a couple cars away.

Over on Platform Six, hissing and moaning, the oldest train in all of Taipei slid into place, and a crowd of passengers shuffled toward it and jumped onto the cars. Sometimes the train had rows of double seats for the romantic types, and sometimes the seats were two rows of benches facing each other. There were never any empty seats. Passengers for Shihlin, Peitou, Kuantu, and Tamsui all used Platform Six for their trains. Among them were people on their way to work, attaché cases in hand, and women with small children in their arms, vendors on their way to the markets to sell specialty items, students holding books or with backpacks on their shoulders, all of them adding color and flavor to the jam-packed cars bound for the northern suburbs of Taipei.

Once the train left Peitou and slowly unrolled on its journey to Tamsui, the scenery outside the windows was nothing short of spectacular. The Tamsui River on the far left, and the buildings that crouched lower and lower, with greater and greater space in between, filled the air with a feeling of sweet nostalgia. The mad tempo of turbulent city life gave way to the soft whine of the accordions played by children in the cabin of the train with mottled walls. The train ride unexpectedly led its passengers on a sentimental journey back to the past. Some of the passengers actually wanted to be imbued with a sense of "long ago," when times had been sweet and good. For them, the train was a tourist site. They sat beside windows and drank in the odors floating up from the river below, they strolled through Tamsui's harbor area to indulge in fish ball soup and watch the sun as it set over the water. Later they would board another train and see the far-off lights of Bali across the river. A bowl or two of fish ball soup was so much easier on the pocketbook than shark's fin soup, and a cinch to enjoy.

However, that train eventually stopped running. The silent banks of the river awaited the construction of the new metropolitan rapid transit systems from the city. Those who longed for old Tamsui times were cut off not only from a lifestyle, but from the fresh country air, too.

During holiday time, throngs of passengers gathered at the ticket windows of the Greyhound bus in both the front and back of the Taipei train station, and at the embarkation points. The Greyhound station was encircled by several wriggling lines that curled like stranded dragons. Taxi drivers stood at the entrance of the station, calling out for customers to pool. Their cars had become obstacles to people arriving at the station, but this obvious violation was never banned. An elderly woman, puffing with exertion and struggling with a large suitcase, threw out curses even as she emerged from between a pair of vehicles that blocked her way. She literally pushed herself into the station. Passengers hurried out through the doors and threw themselves into cabs, waiting for the drivers to pull in travelers in search of a ride.

A young woman appeared beside the cars and began talking prices with a taxi driver. The cabbie took her in as the fourth passenger at a lower than standard price, and slid quickly behind the wheel. Then the taxi roared out in the direction of the expressway.

The roar of the engine roused a baby in the arms of a woman. It wailed so clamorously the woman was in a near-tizzy. She looked for a free corner, plopped down, and pulled out a breast for the child. The little darling sucked in the warm milk, staring all the while at a smudge on the nearby wall with eyes dark and lustrous. When precious baby was finished, it burped. Tiny white bubbles splashed from its mouth onto mommy's pretty coat, and a couple of soft white clouds were imprinted there.

At that time, from every corner of the train station, one could sense indistinct but bothersome odors. The evening breeze sent the putrid stench of the sludge beneath the Chung Hsiao Bridge wafting in the air toward the station, where it ran headlong into the car exhaust, maddening each hurrying individual with perspiration aggravated by the dust stuck to their clothes. The city air turned stifling. The crowds on the buses bounced and wove on a slow trek toward home. The passengers endured each other's odor of sweat that hung in the late afternoon air. They held their breath, and looked forward to a fresh shower or bath at home, free of the shackles of professional or school life, and able to enjoy a private life again!

Restaurants dumped an astounding array of leftovers in the after hours, and homes had more old clothing than they could store. Along with the discarded wrappings of snazzy merchandise, these effused all sorts of scents from all corners of the metropolis.

Eventually the Taipei train station decided to shape up and take on the character of the steel-and-glass high-rises of the city. The station, as the transportation hub of the capital city, should have a metropolitan ambience, should be savvy and sophisticated. With its burgeoning population of millions, the city found a mere six train platforms woefully insufficient. Those platforms were only fit for a city of a few hundred thousand people. The old tracks, like the old roads downtown, should fade into old memories of the prosperous city. This meant future residents could only catch glimpses of old city sights through second-hand information.

Everyone awaited the miracle of transportation to be created by the city. Expectations were high that the days were over when people had to pull cumbersome suitcases up the steps of highway crosswalks, dive down underground walkways, and climb staircases to platform areas. Bruises used to appear on your shoulders where bag straps had strained your blood vessels, and you still only got a ticket for standing room. Only after hours of rocking and swaying did you get to lie flat in your comfortable bed in your hometown, swollen feet propped up high on a couple pillows, sleeping away your fatigue in the shape of a dead body.

Along came huge billows of sand and dust on the square in front of the station. The center hub, with its great construction project, was now off-limits for vehicles. Occasional intruders, failing to be repulsed by the Lane under Construction signs, inevitably ran into One Way Only markers. People drove around like blind gnats groping in the air, taking who knows how many wrong turns, like ships lost in the city. Only directions from passersby could guide them through the twists and turns to their proper destination.

The new train station's appearance gradually began to form as the scaffolding was taken down, revealing the veins of its skin inch by tiny inch like a statue everyone looked up to. Peering through car windows, those who passed the sight every day could appreciate the beauty of the veins. Everyone waited patiently for when the whole façade would be done, and looked forward to the great day the station could stand, proud and brave, basking in the shining rays of the sun.

At the same time, the east side of the city shot up like a fierce dragon. Prosperity was in the air, and tycoons scrimmaged for real estate here to build skyscrapers. A skinny guy who worked as a buyer and seller of old junk and who had eked out a living on the edge of poverty like all of his ancestors had a family of seven living in cramped quarters of only twenty ping—barely more than seven hundred square feet. Next to his shed was the family estate, passed down from generations back, where he piled his old junk, across from a cemetery at some distance. Meanwhile, wind and rain destroyed his pushcart, and rust and deterioration rendered it practically useless. The wheels would hardly turn over the thin asphalt roads.

A big plutocrat came along and promised a huge sum of money. It was so much dough the junk dealer and his wife couldn't count it all even with the aid of all their fingers. His wife had worked every day at a sewing machine at a tailor's, not only supporting herself, but helping the whole family. Was she excited! She grabbed incense sticks and kowtowed her thanks to the ancestors. The husband dashed off in search of old pals for a round of gambling—he would be the banker this time, of course. And the couple started to bicker over money they couldn't lay hands on yet. When old Po-po, the mother of the husband, got wind of the news they were selling the ancestral inheritance, bam! She tumbled just like that into her sickbed. In no time at all, her coughs were hacking like hell, and so horrendous that people all around assumed she'd contracted the latest deadly disease and would spread germs like wildfire.

As innumerable shop lights illuminated the east side of the city, the new train station opened its doors. Trains poured into the dark and shady tunnels deep below the ground. Downsized platforms and the great hall were invaded by misty shadows. Sunrays that once shone on the platforms were now blocked by tall buildings. In front of the new automatic ticket machines, crowds lined up in dragon-sized lines. On dimly lit corridors opened various shops, and people waiting for trains could browse over counters stacked with fancy products, or else they could grab a bite to eat at any number of restaurants. Some people came to the train station just to window-shop.

Young people with comic book characters on their T-shirts couldn't even remember what the old station looked like. Actually, nothing about the new station struck them as so very remarkable. They thought it was totally natural to stroll down aisles with bookstores, chic clothing boutiques, and specialty shops on all sides. But the shops outside the station saw a sharp decline in business. In time, the reputed bookstore avenue gave way to eating establishments, and clothing boutiques were replaced by department stores. The rise of the new train station seemed to have produced a generational divide. Those accustomed to the old station now came up from the shadowy platforms below and couldn't seem to get their bearings amid the entrances and exits marked East, West, South, and North. They just couldn't figure out where to go. But the younger set knew the score. Their steps were quick and sure as they retrieved backpacks from lockers and strode confidently to the designated exits they went through almost every day.

When the construction scaffolding and related paraphernalia were first removed, refined people stopped expecting anything impressive in the new edifice. Those who took a rosier view still believed that a little pizazz would eventually be added to the plain, grayish façade. Only at the grand opening did people accept that the architectural plan simply lacked any distinguishing mark or keynote to catch the eye. No matter your vantage point, the building was such a plain, flat affair, no more than one grayish, shabby-looking cement pillar after cement pillar. Compared to the department stores on the opposite side of the street, the station was like someone without ambition, meeting the transportation needs of the city without swish or swirl. Yet one wondered why, despite its department-store management style, it lacked the drive to put up an attractive appearance. The opinion spread that the hub of transportation for millions of people was missing a keynote. Then the rumor began that the city didn't have a focal point.

But people heading for the train station were not concerned about any of that. They were more concerned about whether the ticket lines would be long, and, if they were in a hurry, they'd occasionally complain, "Why aren't there more ticket vending machines?" They were also interested in the trains staying on schedule. Or, while browsing in station shops, they might suddenly say to themselves, "Uh oh! Did I forget how much time I've got?"

In a city where everything is always changing, peoples' views about transportation, like everything in the atmosphere, are always in a state of flux. Basic truths encouraged people to weigh the value of time and money. The rising cost of train rides, for example, and the misery caused by ten-hour traffic jams on expressways with no place to pull over for a bathroom, drove people to air travel. The rock and sway of city buses, combined with their inexorably poor quality of service, was enough to make a person go out and get a loan for a car, even if they've only been working a couple years. As a result, our roads and by-ways became glutted with cars.

Perhaps the new train station now and again seemed a bit too roomy because so many of its former passengers now drove on their own, but every day there were still so very many people passing in and out of those doors on their way to work or study. Actually, the never-ending increase of cars on our roads was like a tumor spreading in a body. People predicted that one day we would allow so many people to own cars that no land would be left. Those who had entered the city through the old train station and breathed urban air for the first time then had now become the most important part of the city's population. They dispersed into the worlds of education, business, and public service. Some became truly outstanding in our society, and others disappeared into obscurity. It's possible some owned limousines and had no use for the new train station. Others still traveled between the city and their hometown via the station to satisfy their longing for home.

One day a certain gentleman came to the new train station after hosting guests for a fancy dinner. Years earlier, long before his success in the business world, he had arrived in the big city at the old train station with only a simple suitcase in his hand. Remembering how he had raised his eyes at the towering structure before him and determined to go all-out in the city, the rich man approached the new station in his quiet automobile, but he couldn't seem to find the right direction in the maze of lanes circling the station. In the wake of his car, a cloud of dust swirled in the air and silently settled back to the ground. He was still trying as hard as he could to navigate his way into a lane that would take him into the parking lot. The minutes ticked by; in a city grown rich and luxurious, in certain circumstances and moments, people with talent and special achievements and people with common backgrounds, too, suddenly found themselves unable to find a way out in the midst of hordes of buildings.

* From Tsai Su-feng's *Taipei che-chan* 《台北車站》 (*Taipei Train Station*) (Taipei: Linking Publishing Co., 2000).

CHAPTER 5

THE TRAVELS AND LOVER OF A JUNIOR HIGH GIRL

國中女生的旅行與情人

Chung Wenyin 鍾文音

(Translated by Jonathan Barnard 柏松年)

There was someone I wanted to go see: Chen Yu-cheng, an author whom my mother, a writer herself, secretly admired.

I hatched a plan to leave home during winter vacation. After fooling my family that I was going winter camping with the Girl Scouts, I furtively boarded a train. I wanted to travel alone, to see how well I could get along by myself away from home.

I knew Chen wouldn't refuse me—that the greater the challenge to prevailing social mores, the more his interest would be piqued. A young girl coming on her own would appeal to his iconoclastic streak. I was sure of it.

He lived on Taiwan's East Coast, on the shores of the Pacific... You, Chen, were the lusty, elegant savage that I longed to track down and turn into; I wanted you to tell me the secrets of traveling great distances alone, to teach me how to leave home safely and survive.

The Pacific's surf was up and rough. I wanted to scream across the ocean toward the opposite bank, believing that only by so doing could I release my power, push myself across the sea, and find the strength to climb up and walk across the land.

Hualien. Time's mysteries hold dreams in the waves of the Pacific Ocean.

When I was a child, my whole family came here to whale-watch. When I was younger still, the four of us went on a trip to Australia and New Zealand. Over time, the only images of that trip I could recall were of dolphins and whales—and of sheep, getting branded and waiting to be sheared. Or perhaps they were lambs, sacrificial substitutes, bowing their heads and grazing in their pastures, always eating grass or staring dumbly off into the distance, gentle sheep, so easily startled, unaware of the danger so close at hand.

When the dolphins appeared, the water in my range of vision was stained purple by their blood. The whales, their bodies bearing red blooms from the whalers' strikes, would make deep calls. The way to get a mother was to get her child first. Mothers feel a natural duty to protect their children. But when it comes to humans, nature's maternal instinct must be learned. Take my mother: there she was in a Dior suit and high-heeled Valentinos that cost thirty-thousand dollars. Crammed into a small boat with us, her visage wore the expression of a person suffering. When we went diving, my father, older brother, and I were decked out like frogmen—or maybe frog children. My mother, meanwhile, stood on shore, clutching her Chanel bag and worrying that we couldn't see the little diamonds on her red shoes catching the sunlight. She made an effort to shake her head. She was not going in the water.

Her sense of maternal duty had long been wavering. If a whaler had caught me, her trendy clothes, which limited her freedom of movement and desperately required protection, would surely have restrained her. Still a child, I looked at her and suddenly felt hurt: In her eyes I was not nearly so attractive as her tightly clutched purse or the finery she feared would get splashed. I was not the equal of the clothes on her back. Her name-brand possessions had come between us.

Poor Mommy's emotional world had been shattered, but she still had her fashion empire. I believe that my father was just her ATM, and that we were just the happy family photo she could show to the outside world.

I suppose I'm being too harsh. But I can't restrain that attitude, that side of me prone to mockery. I want to join the circus. This life of mine that I'd like so much to avoid is well suited to the clownish prankster.

Once, when we were traveling in Australia, we went for a walk along a riverbed near our hotel and came across a circus camp. A woman, still half-asleep, came out of one of the big circus trucks. The early morning sun lit up her disheveled blond hair. She held a steel cup and brushed her teeth as she walked down to the river. Alongside the truck were lions, tigers, and elephants. To me it looked like a marvelous life.

I tugged at my father's hand to convey my desire to go over and talk to the blond woman. Perhaps she thought it amusing to come across an Oriental child. She splashed some cold water on her face and then turned to speak to me. The strange language struck me as funny, and I laughed and laughed. My father told me that she said she was a tightrope walker.

When we walked to the side of the truck, we saw a poster in which she was wearing white angel wings and perched on swing. In another poster she walked the high wire as tigers and lions paced below.

It was in the midst of this memory that my train pulled into the station.

After I got off, I phoned Chen Yu-cheng. "My name is Lin Tang-shuang," I said, describing myself as that "nu-jen" (which just means "female person") who had asked for his autograph and phone number. Perhaps he remembered? I put special emphasis on the word "nu-jen," thinking that it didn't refer to any specific age.

He said he remembered me but responded with a question of his own: "What do you want, kid?"

I said that I had taken the train to Hualien and was at the station.

"Alone?"

"Uh, could I come and see you? I don't have anywhere else to go. I came especially for you."

"Okay...in that case get on a bus in front of the train station and tell the driver that you want to get off at Jingpu Elementary School."

"Jingtu—clean earth—elementary?"

"No, Jingpu. It's the 'jing' in 'peaceful' and the 'pu' that's the first Chinese character in *Urashima Taro*, the Japanese fairy tale."

"Oh, all right, I'll call you when I get there."

That was the extent of our phone conversation. It was like we were old friends and there was no need for explanations. Why had I come? Why was I alone? Why did I want to see him? There weren't any whys. I think he must have known that starting sans questions would be a marvelous beginning for me. Or perhaps his cool nonchalance was a disguise, and that when I said I was in Hualien all by myself, he felt he couldn't refuse my innocent request to see him. Or maybe he felt that a little girl couldn't be too destructive or belligerent, so he wouldn't worry about letting me come.

First I went to a convenience store near Hualien Station to buy some booze. I was pretty tall and was wearing makeup and grown-up clothes, so I looked eighteen or nineteen. I raised no suspicions buying alcohol and cigarettes. I got a bottle of wine and a bottle of Suntory whiskey, which I had several times seen my English tutor Chuang Mei-huang drinking. Then I bought a carton of Mild Sevens. I felt that giving a whole carton was a powerful gesture.

Once I put the bottles and cigarettes in my knapsack, it became very heavy. It was as if I were carrying my baby to see the child's father. It was amusing to the point of absurdity. I truly didn't know what had possessed me. My father had already grown accustomed to his daughter abandoning him. He said that middle school girls were too complicated and that he never knew what I was thinking. Then he patted my head and took my hand to touch his cheeks, which had grown increasingly rough with age. "In matters of the heart you don't know you have to give back." Then he would let go of my hand, shake his head, and give me some money. My mother would typically shriek about the dangers, the dangers, and then start clipping her nails while listening to a sermon on a cassette, hoping to calm her spirits, which I had agitated.

What a forlorn place the Hualien Train Station is in fall and winter! The summer's tourists have left, replaced with lost souls muttering to themselves. On that day there was a blind man with a cane in one hand and a birdcage in the other; an old man wearing flip-flops and a political campaign baseball cap; a fat woman carrying a plastic bag of detergent; an aborigine chain-chewing betel nuts; a weary-looking pregnant woman; and a young girl, namely me, looking for an escape route—a fifteen-and-a-half-year-old copping a pose and feeling that life all around her was wilting.

Behind me was a sausage stand. The bored proprietor was shooting craps. From an old man's tempura stand nearby wafted an overpowering aroma of overcooked sweetness and decay.

When the bus came, I thought about how my father, ever since I was little, had been accustomed to taking my hand and patting or stroking his face. It was a dreadfully weak gesture from the man of the house. When something bad happened, my mother, on the other hand, would raise her voice, which bore an excruciating resemblance to scratching glass.

Neither of them understood me.

Since I was born, nothing had changed. And how I longed for change! Tell me, Chen—you elegant, poetic wild man of a novelist—tell me your secrets, tell me about your untamed temperament, your views on love and sex, the secret to your being able to set aside your cares and march off to the ends of the earth, about the joys of having sex with countless women. It doesn't bother you, really? Can you truly separate flesh from spirit? I was curious to no end.

The worse-for-wear blue-and-orange plastic chairs stood in their same old places. The sun at two or three in the afternoon slanted across the surface of the plastic, the terrazzo floors, and the pillars finished with small tiles. Resembling wounds, betel nut stains were scattered everywhere. The old man wearing the ugly, cheap campaign cap was smoking. The old woman carrying the plastic shopping bags nagged incessantly. The man suddenly let out a "Fuck!" and followed up by cursing the ruling party and someone's ancestors for eight generations. I watched the scene with great amusement. It was so utterly removed from my hermetically sealed life. Its chaos clashed even more markedly with the immense barren space inside of me. Turmoil and emptiness—they were like twin sisters. I thought I had found my realm, the other side of the sea. From this place to which my father's father—my grandfather—had fled across the Taiwan Strait, his granddaughter would realize his dream of returning to his homeland. Just as he had escaped to this island nation, I would escape from it.

No matter how undignified and hasty, I would replicate that history. I was similar in age to my grandfather when he left mainland China. I would head back to the country that he had abandoned with the mindset of someone who had given up on life.

I was a child who was growing up nourished on travel and geography. I had seen so many films about mainland China—those old clichéd images of sumptuous luxury and homeless peasant wanderers. But I wanted to smell them.

The bus ride offered views of Hualien's coast, of the mountains meeting the sea. I nodded off a few times. On came a blind man carrying a bird, an old aboriginal woman, and two men bearing loads on their backs.

The driver called out Jingpu, and I scurried off and made a telephone call to Chen Yu-cheng. It wasn't long before I saw a small shadow emerge from a small house at the side of the road.

I offered my wine, whiskey, and cigarettes, looking like someone offering oneself for sacrifice.

Delighted with my gifts, Chen said that although I was young, I knew the ways of the world, so he had decided to make an exception and drink with a little kid. Little kid? I screamed. I screamed like my inner wildness had been perceived. In truth I wanted the scream to turn into the howl of a female wolf. He patted my head, and then went to get a bottle opener. Apart from one bowl, one plate, and two or three glasses, his kitchen was empty.

There was also a pile of books and several pieces of clothing. These were the grand sum of his possessions. He said that when he left a place, he never carried away more than a small bag. He didn't feel like bringing anything with him.

Since he couldn't find a corkscrew for the red wine, we drank the Suntory whiskey first. I drank too fast, choking on the first gulp. A burning sensation stung my throat.

"Could I ask some questions?" I inquired. He said that he could tell I was an unusual girl, a very uncommon ninth grader, so he would answer them honestly. Fire away—he'd answer anything.

I recounted my mother and her friends' gossip about him.

With an easygoing manner, he said that he was like the mirror in the Buddhist tale that remained pure and unsullied regardless of the filthy images that flickered across its surface.

Chen Yu-cheng's place leaked water, and it was particularly bad in the bathroom, so I had to wear a farmer's bamboo-leaf rain hat to use the toilet and brush my teeth. As I brushed, I looked in the mirror at the laughable sight of me in the hat. I resembled a fifteen-and-a-half-year-old Vietnamese bar singer who had come to some unfamiliar place for a secret tryst with her lover: pale skin, white clothes, and a farmer's rain hat.

I looked in the mirror, smiled to myself, stuck out the tip of my tongue, sucked in my lips, pulled back the skin near the outer corners of my eyes, and smoothed down the cowlicks in my short hair. Suddenly, I looked up to find that Chen Yu-cheng had appeared in the mirror behind me. Chen said that he wanted to pee. Oh, I said, taking off the hat and handing it to him to put on. As I turned to move toward the door, I heard the wild and powerful sound of his pissing.

I had some improper thoughts, but nothing happened. After he finished urinating, he shook his hips and flushed. Then he gave me back the hat and marched off in his cheap blue flip-flops.

I discovered that I was no Lolita-like seductress, and that he did have thieves' honor. *I wasn't good enough for him*, I thought as I lay in bed. I wished that he would treat me the way he treated all his women. I fantasized about him and then fell asleep. A little girl who had come to the unfamiliar East Coast, to sleep in an unfamiliar bed and breathe unfamiliar air.

The next day he sat on the side of the bed, gently tapped my cheek, and said: "Little girl, time to get up. Let's take a walk by the shore." He sounded like my father—too bad my father never had time to be like that with me.

He told me about the ocean that he looked out upon.

It was where the Hsiukuluan River met the Pacific, a marvel of daily confrontation, ebb and flow, a sonata of give and take.

After listening for a while, all thoughts recede.

A bunch of old women, who looked like mountain ghosts with backs bent at almost ninety-degree angles, descended a knoll. Astonished, I stared at them as they walked, their bodies twisted perversely by time so that they resembled women-chairs. Chen saw me squinting and lost in thought. He said that their hunched backs were probably due to the poor quality of the local water.

It was remarkable how transformed their backs were from the poor water. How, with bodies like theirs, I wondered, could they lie in bed? The first thing they saw would be their feet. What suffering their bodies, bent like chairs at right angles, must have endured! I truly wished that my mother would come and see the fates of other women—take off her expensive shoes, tread barefoot on the earth, and feel the chill or heat.

After Chen heard me slowly retell my experiences in Hualien, New Zealand, and Australia, he said that my mother ought to put down her pen and hand it to me, just as Picasso's father had been stunned at seeing how good a painter Pablo was at an early age and had resolved to stop painting and devote himself to cultivating his son. That peripatetic novelist Chen Yu-cheng really understood me.

A bus stood at the side of the road. Known as keyun—a "guest mover"— it's a tool for transporting passengers. But here it was parked at the side of a coastal road, empty of people. The dirt next to it bore a gob of red juice, its color and moisture content suggesting that it had been left just minutes before as the driver had swaggered off the bus and jerked his head toward the side of the road.

The driver had in fact plunked himself down in a small chair beside a small table in the arcade in front of a small general store across the road. A red-labeled bottle of rice wine on the table provided the scene's only color until a middle-aged woman wearing a dress—a rose pattern over a green field—came out of the store and stole the spotlight. The woman proprietor gave the driver a Tetra-Pak carton of something: "Mix this in and drink." Then she poured herself a glass of the rice wine, added the drink from the carton, and threw a betel nut into her mouth.

Across the road, at the head of a path with a slight incline, two village kids were pushing each other, emitting sounds like broken gongs or the cries of hard-to-tame small animals in heat. Though heard from a distance, the sounds—now high-pitched, now low—still created a dissonance that was hard to bear. Yet the dissonance helped to dispel my afternoon drowsiness.

The sound suddenly ceased. For some unknown reason they had hushed, and their cries had turned into a purely physical language as they punched and kicked each other. Twisted together, faces red and necks swollen and pulsing, half-fighting and half-playing, they appeared for all the world as if they were going to roll off the path and down to the bottom of the gulch. But just then they seemingly negotiated a peace and announced their vagabond knight camaraderie by transforming themselves into a ball of laughter. Their impulsiveness resembled the not-distant waves—the quick back-and-forth, the surprising force as they crashed upon the shore. Several times I had the sensation of watching a drama full of surprising plot twists.

Sitting on a felled tree trunk on the side of the road, I waited lethargically. I pressed my fingers against my temples and then moved down to my jaw. As I pressed on my jaw, I knitted my brow and thought that my tonsils might be infected again. Like my heart, my vulnerable tonsils are always thinking of escape.

I saw Chen Yu-cheng come out of the general store across the street. The proprietor stood up to calculate his bill. Then Chen walked over to me, holding something in each hand. To his right there was still the water that flowed night and day. To his left there was still the small village settlement.

"Feeling poorly?" he asked with concern, seeing my furrowed brow as I massaged my face.

"I didn't sleep well last night." I raised my head, pressed down on both sides of my throat, and uttered a barely audible groan. He squatted and looked at me with interest, his expression conveying silent pity and provocation.

"When there's a sudden rain burst, it's pretty noisy when it hits the corrugated metal on your roof." I said this smiling, then I turned to stare at him, not shrinking back at all. And as we gazed at each other, my hands stopped touching my face in self-pity. I turned my focus to looking into his eyes. He scrunched his eyebrows down as if asking the enemy to surrender, and I said it must be that a little kid like me wasn't enough for him to eat.

"Truly, you're not enough for me to eat," he laughed. "If I was twenty years younger, I might devour you like a wolf or tiger, but now I exist in a strange state," he said.

"What? Are you doubting your own theory about separating spirit and flesh?" I asked.

In the forest, not too far away, you could vaguely see a temple. He didn't respond to my question but rather pointed that way and said, "I've climbed to that temple several times in my leisure. I didn't catch sight of anyone there, but heard chanting and wood clappers." I glanced in the direction of where he was pointing and said that perhaps people were cultivating themselves in seclusion. "In seclusion? In seclusion from what? We ought to call them all to come out."

I thought what he said was funny, and responded, "Haven't you previously done what they're doing? And aren't you sort of doing it now?"

But he was quite serious with his response. He said that he was not in seclusion in the ten years he was in Tamsui, but rather just running back and forth along a few set routes among a few certain women. That was more like retreating to avoid the world. After being alone for a long time, he came to understand loneliness, so that he could go anywhere and be comfortable by himself or in a crowd. "Being part of this mundane world and being outside it are like two sides of the same coin; following one's heart's desire is most important." This is the main point he made.

So my question about separating the spirit from the flesh was now old hat to him, for he could simply do whatever he liked, acting without any qualms. I thought of what he said when we were drinking the night before—that when he hugged a woman goodbye in the train station it was like they were glued together. But once she was on her train, he could turn right around, call up another, and shack up at her house for many days. Wandering, his heart was carefree.

This was the freest being that I, as a junior high school student, had yet encountered. Chen's life had completely entranced me, because its qualities were so different from the upper-middle-class circles I traveled in, so different from the values my parents had taught me. He clearly and honestly uncovered his deepest layers for me to see.

Smiling, he looked at me empathetically and swung what he was carrying into my hands. As I looked at what had been transferred into my hands, it was my turn to have an odd expression on my face. It was like a familiar object stirring a sense of recollection. Inside the plastic bag he gave me was a Kekounaitzu coconut cookie, a pastry twist, and a can of Assam tea.

"Where is Assam?" I duly asked.

"In India," he said. Then he waved his hands and spoke about distant India.

"Why don't we go together?" I suddenly blurted out.

He burst out laughing and both corners of his mouth turned way up. I had never seen him laugh like that; it was like some wild call. "Going with you wouldn't be safe."

"Not safe?" I hit him with a cookie.

"Yeah, you're body and mind full of some strange desire to be an adult. You'll tempt me to commit a crime." Chen sat on a stool and plucked a weed. The gray sea in front of him climbed into his eyes, and he suddenly sighed and said slowly, "Young lady, when I look at you, it's like seeing my youth, my long-departed dreamlike youth."

Back when an adolescent named Chen was a pale boy hanging out in the West Gate section of Taipei, he could totally distinguish between the spirit and the flesh, love and desire. The world was chaotic; the body was pure. Fucks for fucks, dreams for dreams. When he awoke, he was feverish; when he was doing it, he was muddle-headed. When he finished, he'd be lost—before once again throwing himself into the tide of humanity and not knowing where he'd end up, and then once again entering a twisted state, coming and going.

As long as you cast a line from shore, someone would take the bait. There were encounters with strangers' bodies, entwinings and couplings in the dark, then separations without feeling. The young Yu-cheng walked the streets alone, a floating spirit nimbly passing through cracks in the crowd.

He said that in those pale days of emptiness he was like a candle in the wind. It was for that reason that he started working out. By training his body, he'd also be training his spirit. That was the state I saw him in, as big and strong as a bear. It was the first time that I had known a man with a body like a bear and a soul like silk.

Finally, he said that he hoped that I wouldn't talk about my visit to him. I regarded his reminder as a slight and was somewhat displeased.

"Are you unhappy?"

"No."

About an hour later the keyun bus came, and I got on. Apart from me, the passengers included another blind man carrying a bird, an aborigine constantly sipping rice wine, and a tired woman carrying a chintz bag.

I took a window seat and stuck my face out the window. Chen's face was on my right. The ocean breeze had blown his frizzy, shoulder-length hair into two short, fat wings. He wore solid black clothes, glasses, and cartoon-character flip-flops that clashed with his literary air. Printed on them in English was the phrase "I love you." I looked at him with amusement.

As the bus started moving, Chen's black clothes became a small dot and then disappeared. I imagined him returning to where he lived and, as night fell, smashing open the bottle of red wine to drink alone. I opened the package of coconut cookies, breathed in their sweet aroma, and started eating them. The surging Pacific Ocean still raged on my right. This was the first time I had ever traveled alone, the first time I had slept in a man's bed. Nothing had happened, and yet everything had happened. In my mind he was my first lover.

I couldn't bring myself to finish off the coconut cookies. When I returned home, I stashed them in a desk drawer, where they remained until Chinese New Year, when I heard my mother's sharp cry, and the cookies and a colony of ants were deposited with a swoosh into the garbage.

Afterward, this was the only kind of cookie I ate. It was an act of faithfulness by a junior high school girl, a secret kept from her first travels alone. Believe me when I say that I am more faithful than any of you and better able to keep my mouth sealed tight.

> * From *Chiu-shih-san nien san-wen hsuan* 《九十三年散文選》 (*Collected Essays, 2004*), ed. Chen Fang-ming 陳芳明 (Taipei: Chiu Ko Publishing, 2005).

CHAPTER 6

BABY, MY DEAR

親愛的小孩

Marula Liu 劉梓潔

(Translated by Chris Wen-chao Li 李文肇)

1. POPCORN

I want to have a baby.

   You'll get over it. That's how a bunch of childless girlfriends past the ripe old age of forty put it to me. They, too, were once taken with the irresistible urge to have a baby in their early thirties, to the point where the bell-like laughter of every babbling two-year-old they saw on the subway would bring them to tears. But it's just the hormones talking, telling you that it's now or never, and once you get over it then it'll all be fine. They give me a pat on the back and tell me that once I'm over it I can return to the carefree life of smoking, drinking, meeting new men, and traveling the world—what's not to like?

Yes, it's the hormones sounding the alarm bells, like a dedicated restaurant server courteously hovering by your side, reminding you that it's time for last orders, asking whether you would like anything else from the kitchen. You shake your head, sipping your red wine, firm in the belief that you are here only to drink—that is, until your stomach starts churning. You wave him over, only to have him tell you with an apologetic look that the kitchen has closed for the night. Through the glass partition behind the bar you see the kitchen assistants ready with mop and detergent. What a letdown. The server or the bartender, by chance, feeling sorry for you, passes you a few kernels of popcorn. But you are perfectly aware that as you slip these vacuous little cloud-shaped bites into your mouth, you'll be staring with envy at the folks in the booth next to you, their table piled high with tortillas, cheese fries, buffalo wings, double pepperoni pizza, chocolate soufflé, and macadamia nut-dressed vanilla ice cream—like an endless smorgasbord that grows all the more sumptuous as the crowd erupts in cheers and laughter. How you wish you could bring your knife and fork to their tableside and ask, mind if I dig in?

No, you don't want to sink to that level.

The carefree life of smoking, drinking, meeting new men, and traveling the world, to me, is like a box of popcorn teetering on its edge, ready to topple at any moment and scatter its contents across the floor. I don't have it in me to pull it off, growing into a forty-something career woman bereft of husband or child, yet proud of being a looker and a mover-and-shaker. No, without a child, I'd be hunched on the ground trying to pick up the scattered pieces.

Once I'm over it, things are not going to be fine. When I'm over it, I'll be done, for good.

2. A Sex Life

To not have a sex life and pine after a child is as ludicrous as not buying a lottery ticket yet dreaming of winning the jackpot. But before we go there, let me recount the previous lots that I've been dealt in this facet of life, a sex life in which, like with my hand at the lottery, I seem to win a little and lose a little, like buying a two-dollar payslip only to win two dollars, again and again in a never-ending cycle. There were times, my little baby, when it seemed as if I was ever so close to having you.

It happened on my thirtieth birthday—I was scheduled to fly to San Francisco that very evening. H was kind enough to use what brief lunch break senior managers are afforded these days to take me out. Luggage in tow, I rushed to his city by high-speed rail, where, as always, he was waiting for me at the station entrance. As I stepped out, there he was, in the sharpest of suits, leaning against his car, smiling blandly and waving to me. After lunch at a high-end Italian establishment, he chaperoned me back to the station, where I sneaked my hands into the sleeves of his linen-blend suit and rubbed against him, using all my womanly charms to bring to his attention that my flight wasn't until five in the afternoon. He appeared wise to my tactics, but did his part to fight temptation. I touched him some more, and whispered that I was in my safe period. I was sure he would want nothing more than to stop the car and hold me in a tight embrace, but instead he remarked in all seriousness, "I have a meeting in another half-hour at three—if only you had said something earlier, we could have skipped lunch."

You've got to be joking—if only I had said something earlier? Like what? Like telling him back at the station that I had brought two burgers from Mos Burger, so we could go to a motel room and celebrate the funkiest thirtieth birthday ever? I had the urge to tell him that if sex was on his mind he shouldn't be such a jerk, but could not bring myself to do so. Instead I stared at him with lovestruck puppy-dog eyes and traced little circles on his biceps.

We circled the station looking for a spot, wading through a landscape of vacant spaces and construction sites. The roads, dotted with newly erected office blocks, were freshly paved and saw little traffic. He stopped in front of an overgrown lot and asked, "How's here?" How he was able to come up with so many sun shades and window blinds without as much as getting out of the driver's seat I did not know, but in a matter of seconds he was able to fully shield the car's interior from external view, like an expert outdoorsman pitching a tent in the wild. Perhaps with the push of a button even the license plate would cover itself up. He took off his pants and I removed my blouse. He ordered me to recline the seat fully so that the seatback would be level. He then climbed over and pressed down on me. Who would have guessed he'd turn out to be the king of car sex? I was not turned on though, but instead felt cheap, like a pay-by-the-hour whore accosted by a tech industry executive eager for a quickie out in the bush before returning home to the wife and kids. I just wanted it to be over with. H, gentleman that he was, always made a point of seeing me come before he did. So I faked an orgasmic moan, after which he upped the tempo and duly let out a manly grunt of satisfaction. He delivered his load—fully inside of me.

Dragging my luggage, I retreated into a stall in the ladies room at the high speed rail terminal and sat there for a good while, reminiscing about the first time we were intimate, which was in a posh boutique hotel with a tub the size of a double bed; the second time was at my apartment, where the foreplay included dessert on the balcony set to candlelight. Today would be the third time—on a nondescript lot in the middle of nowhere that someday might turn into a commercial warehouse or a luxury mansion—who knows? I knew only that I desperately needed a shower. I looked around me and only wished the toilets here had hoses extending from the water tanks, the way they do in certain Southeast Asian countries. Oh well. It looked like I was going to have to carry his seed with me to San Francisco, on my birthday that is. We'd fly across the International Date Line, where, in San Francisco, it'd still be my birthday, and that, my little baby, would be the day of your conception.

The next few days, as I made my rounds of Fisherman's Wharf, the Golden Gate Bridge, City Lights Bookstore, Café Coppola, Haight-Ashbury, the Castro, and Napa Valley, I couldn't help but think of you, my dear baby, about how, if you were really there in the waiting, what a fabulous first trip this would be to the mecca of hippiedom. Would you grow up to be a flower child? I would check my email at the public terminals of the hotel lobby each morning, but no word from H—not that I would want to write him either. A week later I am back in Taipei. He hadn't called, and I refused to call him—or so I put up a pretense until days later when I finally gave in. He didn't pick up, and never called back.

Another two days and I got a letter: *You are a wonderful girl who deserves to go in search of the happiness you truly deserve.* What a load of bull! And yet, there I was, frozen in front of the computer screen the entire morning crying away. Oh, and as it turns out, I was not pregnant. Soon after, though, along came my second lottery ticket in the form of L.

Our paths first crossed in the spirituality section of a bookstore, where we conversed in simple English on topics ranging from yoga and new age to Osho and India. He concluded our little banter with the remark, "Great talking to you, have a good day," and I said, "You, too," and with that we went our separate ways. But a good hour or half-hour later, as I was stepping out of the bookstore, there he was, with his back to the door, looking out onto the street like he was waiting for something or someone. No, it wasn't a cab or a friend or anything one could easily put into words that he was hoping to catch, but something more amorphous, more ephemeral, more enigmatic. That all-too-familiar look of loss and disorientation, as if searching for the one, I know it all too well because I've been there, too—only the object of my quest has always eluded me.

I walked up to him and bid a friendly good-bye, and he responded with a smile and a cursory nod. As I turned and headed for the subway, he ran up to me and asked, "Want to come to my place?" I said, "Okay."

We hopped in a cab and ended up at a residential suite of the type rented out to foreigners on short-term assignment in Taipei. We then undressed, copulated, showered, clothed ourselves, and walked downstairs to the nearest intersection, where we said good-bye for real and went our separate ways. All was transacted in a little under an hour. It was already sundown when I entered his apartment, and now it wasn't even dark.

The duration of the sex was really a joke: doggy-style, missionary position, ejaculation, and done—like rolling out a sandwich on a fast-food assembly line. There was no hugging or kissing as we both strove to maintain a single point of contact between our two bodies. I was handed a freshly laundered crisp white towel before entering the shower, and after I had dried myself it was duly tossed into the wash. He himself later used a different towel. It resembled the kind of service you would expect at a spa (or perhaps at a makeshift massage parlor staffed by the blind). As I exited the shower room, I found him nude on the balcony looking out. I approached him from the rear and gave him a bear hug. He reached behind him with his hands and squeezed my buttocks through the towel.

In the elevator he told me that, despite appearances, this wasn't the kind of behavior he normally engaged in. He also lent me two books of his, even though I had the feeling it wouldn't matter in the least if I did not return them. Even if we were to never see each other again, all would be fine. But that wasn't how things turned out. The next few months or so, I would get a text message from him every two or three weeks, and we would meet up to repeat the very same behavior all over again.

L was a stickler for using protection—having backpacked through India, Thailand, Indonesia, and now Taiwan, and sampled the various women along the way, it was the least he could do to ensure hygiene and personal courtesy—for which reason I never bothered to worry about whether I would be mother to a blond-haired, blue-eyed Eurasian baby.

L couldn't keep it up for very long, which made it frustrating when it came to removing the condom, by which time he had long gone soft. I complained about this to my BFF Mori, who could divine the appearance of a man's member just by gazing at his mug. Mori had long wanted me to send him a photo of L to see if there was hope yet, at which moment it dawned on me that I didn't even know the man well enough to take a picture of the two of us cheek-to-cheek with my smartphone. Like delivering a physics lecture, Mori explained to me that when material is of the same density, the more oblong the object, the lesser its rigidity. Given that Europeans are better endowed when it comes to length, the subsequent reduction in stiffness is to be expected. In other words, if you gain a little here, you're bound to lose a little there—that's how I see it anyway—the lesson being that life oftentimes is a zero-sum game.

On one occasion the pack of condoms that L had bought was, for some reason, impossibly difficult to tear open. Now don't all condoms come in three-packs? Why is it that every time he's having sex with me he's having to open a new pack? What happened to the other two? I dare not ask—not that such a question would lead anywhere. The only reasonable explanation is that he must have used them (he could, of course, tell me that he lent them to a neighbor—if anyone would believe such a lame excuse). Does it bother me? I'd be lying if I were to say it didn't—why else would I be sitting here stark naked watching him writhe and squirm, without as much as an empathetic "Sweetheart, is there anything I can do?" Yes, there's a dark side of me that wants to just sit idly by and watch him slowly go soft—a kind of silent revenge —not that it would do me any good.

He picked up a paring knife from the kitchen sink and angled it to pierce through the stubborn packaging, only to see it slip and gouge his palm. Blood started to gush from the center of his hand. No longer fixated on whether he would go soft, I rushed over to tend to his wound. The wound was small but deep. I grabbed a wad of tissues and ordered him to apply pressure. We scrambled into our clothes and hailed a taxi to the nearest hospital, where he ended up with two stitches. Soon we were on a cab ride home, happy as two little children who had just survived the biggest of scares. As if still short of breath, he asked, "So what did you tell the doctor about how I hurt myself?"

"You were shelling an oyster," I said, giggling like a schoolgirl, and asked him, "What did the doctor say?"

"The doctor said," he repeated, "'Oyster shells can be nasty, you really got to be careful!'" We laughed hysterically, oblivious to the people around us. "A real genius, you are!" he exclaimed. He put his arm around my shoulder and kissed me on the forehead. God knows if the cab driver was thinking I was the kind of woman who trawled the nightclubs to pick up foreign men. I was not, of course—I just picked up whatever came my way.

Back at L's place, we ended up having sex after all. And that was the only time he let me stay the night. He let me rest my head all night on the hand that wasn't wrapped in gauze, but it was hardly a watershed moment. Two months later, he left Taipei for Europe. "Bon voyage," I texted. I was in a crowded subway compartment at the time, standing next to the door, where I could see my sorry reflection in the glass. I arrived at my stop but did not go home, instead crossing over to the opposite platform to catch an inbound train to Mori's joint.

Mori had a new partner—Yoo was his name. His old partner went by the name of Kirk. Now Kirk was a master mixologist who specialized in mixing up cocktails to perfectly capture the fantasies of the customer, be it abstract melancholy musings about a past lover, or visualizations as specific as heartthrob Bae Yong Joon making a house call at four in the morning to service your A/C. What became of Kirk, I did not ask. Mori waved me in and told me Yoo would make me whatever I fancied. Something with a sour kick, I told him. I told Mori if it turned out I was pregnant with a Eurasian child, I might as well give it up to him and Yoo to adopt. Mori understood I was in one of my moods, and stepped out from behind the counter with arms open. "Come on, let's have a hug."

"Why, Mori, you queer bastard, why is it that you're always able to hit me in my soft spot?" As he placed his big fat palm over my forehead, tears started streaming down.

He told me, "Yoo is psychic, you know; why don't you ask him what the future has in store?"

I wiped away my tears and said, "Okay, let's ask him when I'm going to have a baby."

Something of an introvert, Yoo stared straight into my eyes for a few seconds, then looked down, like he was receiving transmissions from another world. He then looked up, "You know, there is a little boy with big, round eyes following you around, waiting for you to bring him into this world."

"Like, where?" I asked, looking all around me.

"Oh, he's here alright," Yoo assured me, "and has always been."

I'd actually been told the same thing by Big Daddy, who says that when a baby wants to come into this world, he will find a way—there is no stopping him. The important thing is that love be present the instant daddy and mommy consummate their union. If love can be sensed, the baby will want to come.

Oh yes, love. So when daddy and mommy were messing around on a deserted lot by the railway station, or when daddy had to get two stitches from trying to tear open a pack of condoms and mommy was sitting by laughing hysterically, you must have felt disgusted and must not want to have anything to do with us. Is that what it is, my dear little baby?

3. THE WORD

Love. What is love? Can it be teased apart from sex? And how do you tell if a man truly loves you, or if he is in it only for the sex? Questions such as these, along with how to achieve instant orgasms and how to make your man cry out in ecstasy, can be found in the magazine *Cosmopolitan*, where you'll find articles written by experts and personality quizzes designed to measure your every sexual propensity—hardly anything new, but I read every issue in the hair salon. And here I am again, bombarding Mori with a battery of questions, as if I were some human incarnation of a personality test. So, the way H likes to hold my hand when he's driving, is that a sign of love? And when I'm engrossed in reading, L likes to reach over and sweep my bangs to the side—is that love?

Across the bar, a mature babe with long, thick fake eyelashes flashes me a look of disbelief, then smiles and says, "Girl, you want to know if you really love a man? It all comes down to this: Are you willing to swallow his load?"

"Whoa, lady, that is wild!" By that standard I've never really been in love before. (Well, there was this one time when L and I toyed with the idea, but I ended up vomiting over the toilet. How so very embarrassing!)

Truth be told, I'm just feigning ignorance. I know all too well whether love is present. All becomes clear at the moment of parting.

I had been sleeping with N on and off for some two years without ever having broached the subject of love. It wasn't until three days before he was on a plane bound for Los Angeles that he told me he was emigrating with his family and would never return. He had some books of mine, he said, and was asking whether he should bring them over or if I wanted to go and fetch them (How civil a breakup—he might as well have suggested dispatch by courier service). I ended up going over to his place. At the time I was renting a room in a poky apartment, and would go over to his fully equipped one-bedroom suite once a week, where the private bath and full kitchen seemed like such a luxury. Now all that was left was a long sofa and a sack of books awaiting my pickup. We sat at the two ends of the sofa with barely a word to say to each other. We met two years ago at a house party at his place. As the guests were filing out—some putting on their shoes and others already queuing at the elevator—I was still bent over struggling to get into my wrap-around sandals, at which point he said to me, "You, stay." I listened, and sat back onto the couch, waiting for him to see everybody off. And that was how it all started.

There were some dishes left on the kitchen shelf. "You want to take these?" he asked, as if struggling to find the right words for a tender farewell.

I shook my head as two pearly dewdrops rolled from the corner of my eye. My gaze fixated on the white floor tiles, I told him, "Just say the word, and I can drop everything and be on the next plane with you to the States." I looked up and saw two streams of tears on his cheeks. We stared each other in the eye, and he pulled me into his embrace, telling me, "You're still young, you know, life still has much in store for you." He walked me to the door, caressed my left cheek, and said, "Be happy, okay?"

I repeated, "Just say the word, and I'll come with you." That was probably the bravest I've ever been in this life.

He ultimately left, after which I signed up for a flurry of yoga classes from beginning to advanced covering different schools and sects and eventually succeeded in shedding several pounds. Then it dawned on me that there was something odd about the sequence of events. I asked around and discovered that while N was seeing me he had a steady girlfriend known to all, and it was with her that he emigrated to the US.

N would occasionally write me from stateside, attaching funny video clips, cute animal photos, or forward accounts of horrific abuses perpetrated by fast food chains. And I would reply with lame one-liners (I never dared ask why he cried those tears the night we parted), if only to keep in touch, to convince myself that such a person still existed in this world. Two years went by. I would occasionally see H, and then L, and then the two would again exit from my life.

So what am I trying to say? That my past relationships have been traumatic, and that is why I've subjected myself to this emotional exile? No, that is not how it is at all. Love, as it happens, is not governed by the law of cause and effect. Every time a new love interest appeared, I would hope that it would be the beginning of a steady, long-term relationship that I could tell all the world about, and that we could have a baby and live happily ever after. And yet, like putting things into a pocket that is torn, everything that comes into my life seems to eventually slip away.

In love we don't always reap what we sow, yet, time and again, life finds a way to fill the gaps between relationships. Two days after L departed, I got a text from N asking whether I wanted to spend the New Year holidays in the States. It was hardly the ending I was hoping for, and I kept telling myself this was no more than another lottery gamble, but I booked my pricey air ticket without a second thought. N checked us into a bed-and-breakfast in a Chinese suburb of L.A. and stayed with me the whole time, never once returning home. On New Year's Eve we crossed the border into Tijuana, then drove to Las Vegas for a week of fun and feasting, followed by a trip into the desert, where we spent the night in a wood cabin in the Mojave National Preserve before returning to the City of Angels. But other than sleeping in the same bed, our behavior was more like that of two friends: shopping at warehouse stores and designer outlets, going to bars and restaurants, and gambling at the blackjack table, where the staff would inquire with typical American bubbliness, "Are you newlyweds? Do you have kids?"

And, as if of one mind, we would both respond, "No, we're just friends."

Can't remember which night it was—we'd had sex in the dark and were holding each other in a tight embrace when I started coming to tears and begging him to have a baby. "I'll raise him myself," I said, "you won't have to do a thing—I'll even put it down in writing." But he refused, saying it was a responsibility and mental burden he wasn't ready to bear, and that I was being too simplistic and naive. "I would love our baby so, so much," I told him, and then let burst the floodgates like the whole world had wronged me, crying myself to the point where even I found myself repulsive, and then I eventually cried myself to sleep. In a hazy stupor halfway through the night, I sensed his member enticing me, wanting to have a second go at it, and my body responded in kind. But at the climax he pulled out as usual, and shot a full load of cum onto my belly. It occurred to me to go to the bathroom and use my fingers or a wad of tissues to scoop up the semen and deliver it into my system. Who knows if some miracle might happen? In the tabloids you read about people getting pregnant from swimming in a public pool. But I was overcome with lethargy, unable to lift my eyelids, bound to the bed by the many traces of tears and strands of dried semen. Wave after wave of fatigue and drowsiness pushed me into ever deeper stages of sleep, where I began to heal. It was daylight when I woke up. N was already up, fully dressed and sitting beside the window. I sat nude between the soft white sheets, quietly admiring his silhouette against the morning light. He turned to look at me with tenderness in his eyes and offered to go get coffee from downstairs.

On the final day of our tryst, he drove me to the airport. We parked in the passenger loading zone and he helped me offload my luggage. Parting had never been his forte, as he didn't take well to hugs and kisses, so I flashed a toothy smile and said good-bye, and, luggage in tow, turned to leave.

He reached and placed his hands on my shoulders, then whispered in my ear, "Be happy now."

I never looked back, but instead headed straight for the departure hall, went through the most stringent of airport security screenings, and duly boarded my plane. On the fourteen-hour flight back, where service typically included three full meals, I refused to eat a thing, nor did I read or watch feature films. Instead, I just wrapped my arms around my shoulders and slept through the entire ordeal. Upon landing, the Southeast Asian cutie in the next seat offered me chewing gum, but I turned him down. It had become all too clear that the biggest lesson from this trip was that I had come back empty-handed, and that there would be no more lottery tickets for me to scratch. Okay, so the metaphor sucks, I know, but what I am trying to say is that it had dawned on me that I could no longer cry to my girlfriends like some naive little child, whining about relationships that seemingly lead nowhere, or pretend that I was playing the field. Instead, I needed to face the facts. And the facts of the matter are that I am a pathetic little bitch appreciated by no one and desired by no one.

How cruel it is not to be loved. But would you cry to a slot machine that has taken all your money, tearfully falling to your knees, pleading with it and asking why the sudden cruel treatment when all seemed perfectly fine yesterday? You wouldn't, would you? What it comes down to is that you had to be eager and willing in the first place.

There is no point in griping over not receiving something of equal or greater value than what you put in, for no one put a gun to your head. You can only blame your luck. Blame the fact that you are a miserable bastard.

From this point on, this miserable bastard ceased to have a sex life.

4. T<small>HE</small> F<small>ERTILITY</small> C<small>ULT</small>

Papa Che and Mama Che are the ringleaders of our local fertility cult. They had been together fifteen years prior to marriage, during which time they trekked through every known mountain range in Taiwan, tracing rivers and streams to their sources. As if that weren't enough, upon graduation they followed the act with a trip to the Americas, where they scaled sheer ice cliffs in Colorado and made their way up the highest peak in Argentina. Papa Che ultimately achieved his dream of climbing the Seven Summits. As he returned with his team following their conquest of Mount Everest, Mama Che went to pick him up at the airport, and there, in front of a swarm of reporters, he went down on his knees and asked for her hand in marriage. Before they had time to plan a wedding, though, the two went on a honeymoon to Paris and Barcelona, and when they returned, Mama Che was with child. They decided to name their baby Che, after Che Guevara.

"If he was conceived in Spain and Paris, why not just call him, well, Spenis?" I asked, instantly breaking into a chuckle, as did Mama Che, whereas Papa Che shouted from the adjacent study, "If his name is Spenis, I should hate to think what nickname the kids at school would give him!" And we lost ourselves in laughter. Bottle in hand, ten-month-old Baby Che frolicked in the little space between his mother and me, giving out a giggle like the ring of silver bells.

Papa Che and Mama Che were my best buddies in college. Their life's ambition was to travel the world, or so it seemed until you got to know them better. You'd see that road tripping is something they did on the side while they won prestigious scholarships to study abroad and earn doctoral degrees (Papa Che will tell you that you've got it the other way around, that touring is their life's calling while the studying part is incidental). Now that they are back from their sojourns, they have bought a house and car in the perennially sunny climes of Southern Taiwan, where they hold teaching posts and raise their delectable child. What a picture-book existence! Whereas my attempts at pursuing advanced degrees abroad are patchy at best, not to mention my tattered love life. What have I achieved in all these years? I guess you could say that I've managed to hold on to my freedom.

Ah, yes—freedom. I remember the Ches used to return from abroad every once so often and summon the old posse, now scattered in different parts of the island, to regroup in Southern Taiwan, where we would drink beer and chomp on seafood in view of the sunset at Siziwan Bay, then lie in a row on the sea wall at Sun Yat-sen University. There, brushed by the ocean breeze, one of the guys would play his guitar while the rest of us sang to the melodies of Bobby Chen. Oh those beloved lines—"Say goodbye to the crowded paradise," and "I want you, freedom, like a bird."

But now they've finally settled down, and I too have become more available, no longer ditching my friends for potential dates. They would often invite me over, and I would hop on a high-speed train to their southern port and join them on their family outings. Little by little, I watched Baby Che grow to six months, ten months, a year old, a year-and-a-half, two years, and then learn to crawl, learn to walk, learn to run, learn to say Mama, Papa, learn to say Aunty, learn to say thank you and good-bye. Then Mama Che went on to carry her second child. I watched her go through her first trimester, second trimester, third trimester. We no longer frequent the windswept seaside and play guitar, but instead take the toddler shopping at big box stores. With time the Ches see that I have a gift for looking after children, and are content to leave baby and cart to my care while they hunt down Australian short ribs, Italian gourmet cheeses, and French country wines of manga renown. I sing the baby silly songs, talk to him in baby-speak, and take him to the different aisles and refrigerated chests to show him various food items. "Now this is a fishy—do you want a fishy, Little Che? And this is milky milky. Did you drink your milky milky today?"

As the couple returns with an armload of merchandise for the shopping cart, I am asked by Papa Che how my internship in single motherhood is progressing so far. "Ring, ring, we have a winner," I say. And Little Che repeats after me, "Ring, ring. Ring, ring."

We return to the sumptuous Che residence, complete with robotic vacuum and automated dishwasher. As dinner is prepared, other members of the cult arrive on the scene. Papa John and Mama John show up with two-and-a-half-year-old Little John, who, together with two-year-old Little Che, empties a box of toys onto the floor and starts making the grunts and noises of little animals. As they stomp and strut around the place like it is their own tropical jungle, the adults are engrossed in their own form of amusement, waving their wine glasses and getting ready to listen to the ringleader preach his sermon.

"You have got to have a baby, even if it means a life of single motherhood." This was Papa Che's habitual opening line.

"Give it another two years," I say, "by then I'll be more secure financially."

"We're not talking about planting flowers here," says Papa Che, "You don't just plant a seed and expect it to sprout the next day—you really have got to draw up some backup plans."

"Like it's that easy," I retort, "This is not Denny's—you don't just fry an egg and then set it aside for later use."

"Oh, by the time you're forty," says the ringleader, "you'll have tried all there is to try and seen all there is to see—what are you going to do then if you don't have a child? Fly to outer space?"

"Oh, you never know," I say, "maybe I'll cook it up with an astronaut!" It's all crazy talk, I know, but no crazier than the time Mama John had a bit too much to drink and announced with fanfare that she would never regret having Little John, even if her marriage were to fall apart. Papa John almost dropped his glass.

No regrets at all. I know of a few other friends who had originally planned on staying single all their life, who were then saddled with an unplanned pregnancy and opted to keep the child, embarking on a path of pacifiers, diapers, cribs, and strollers, making do with under three hours of sleep a day and putting up with wine of the bargain basement variety—and yet they have no regrets. Time and again, when I left my cult meeting and headed north on a high-speed bullet train, there would be a screaming baby in the carriage or obnoxious little children turning the place upside down. Yet with time I've learned to be patient with them— no longer am I the grim-faced scary lady giving them a hard time. These monthly internships in motherhood have softened my rough edges and turned me into a more tolerant soul. Little baby, my dear, if it weren't for you, chances are I'd go on hurting people and hurting myself with these uncurbed excesses of my personality.

Big Daddy is not big on children, but he believes in finding a partner. "You've got to have a partner before you can even think of having a baby," he says. Big Daddy is my mother's age, a good twenty-four years my senior, making us both monkeys in the Chinese zodiac. His son is also a monkey, but a good twenty-four years younger. Having wanted a child for the longest time, he finally got his wish in his forty-eighth year. By now he very much has his own theory of fertility and conception: If a child wants to come into this world, he will find a way, but to facilitate his arrival you will need to find a good partner. I snap back like a spoiled teenage daughter, I'd much rather go on spring break in Bali, and choose not to know whether the child in my belly is black, white, Asian, or Latino until the moment he comes out of my snatch! Scary, he says, but he knows full well that when I have my mind set on something, there is no stopping me.

And I really went, but nothing came of the trip. I would hang out in front of the busiest café in the mountain resort of Ubud, where local young men with rocking bods would sit in a row and casually inquire of passers-by whether they were looking for company. And like the most squeamish of prudes I would quickly walk away. I did see some Western and Asian women traveling alone who took them up on their offer. I have no idea how much it cost or how the business was transacted, but one day at the bus stop, I saw an Indonesian hottie holding the hand of a pudgy, pale-skinned Korean woman, telling her, email me, okay? The woman gave him a rub on the cheeks. I'm thinking, maybe this woman is carrying in her belly a mixed-race Indonesian-Korean child— why is it that she can and I cannot? What am I so picky about? What a price to pay for my pride! Mori used to tell me to go to him if I ever needed a man to father my child. He says there is no shortage of rock 'n' roll anarchist-types at his bar who are all too happy to sleep around like dogs. They would bring their gear to his joint, busk in exchange for booze, and then spend the night in one of his booths—surely they wouldn't mind helping out an older gal with aspirations of motherhood— maybe you could tip them twenty dollars so they would have money to buy breakfast. Yeah, yeah.

Occasionally, on a random street corner, I would spot the man of my dreams, tall and suave like a Korean supermodel, and immediately text Papa Che and the gang. "Target identified. What to do now?"

"Hop in bed, of course!" reads Papa Che's reply.

Yeah, right. I can hardly bring myself to speak to the guy, let alone get into bed with him. But I know full well this is not my style—I'm just messing around. Deep down I know that Big Daddy is right, that ultimately I will need to find love, that love needs to be present the moment a man and a woman consummate their union. After all, we do live in the twenty-first century—what modern woman would be content to just shut her eyes and spread her legs, enduring the pain of unpleasurable sex just so that a child could be brought into this world? What would be the point?

Which is why, for the remainder of my stay in Bali, I all but confined myself to a yoga studio situated amidst acres of rice fields, where we would chant, meditate, exercise, and focus on breathing. Mori has some unkind things to say about yoga studios. These new age workshops, he says, are the haunt of divorcées, widows, and losers—don't you go off the deep end now, don't turn into one of them. Well, I've come to terms with the fact that I am a loser in love. The other day, as the master healer was leading a recitation of my favorite prayer, "Lokah Samastah Sukhino Bhavantu," I began to sob uncontrollably. The verse roughly translates to "May happiness and freedom be upon all sentient beings of this world." I chant the holy words again and again, bringing deliverance to the many men who have passed on me, in the process also delivering myself from suffering.

5. The Little Boy

I catch an early morning flight back to Taiwan, and see a text from the ringleader waiting for me the instant I power up my phone. "Ahead 2-0 now. Get your act together, girl!"

So Mama Che gave birth to her second child three days ago. She sends me a series of clips, which I click and view as I wait by the baggage carousel. So this is Sister Che at three days, a refined version of Baby Che! That puny nose and tiny mouth, those big bright eyes wandering in every which direction, as if so eager to explore the world around her, that cute little yawn that makes me want to melt!

I text back and say, "Your girl is adorable! I want to have a baby boy to woo her when they grow up," and end the message with a string of kisses.

Charged with positive energy—not sure whether from the stay in Bali or from the birth of the baby girl, I break my habit of heading straight for the sack, and instead take an airport bus to a department store to pick out a present for the newborn. There is barely any foot traffic, as the store had only just opened, making it my favorite time to shop. Before heading upstairs to kids' apparel, I make my rounds of the fragrance therapy section, comparison shopping at different beauty counters before finally returning to the first.

The young counter clerk, eager to serve me, assumes the tone of an acquaintance and asks if I want to try their eucalyptus essential oil. "It clears up the respiratory tract," he says, "and is great for children."

"Children? But I don't have any children," I protest, as I tug slightly on my oversized cotton-linen blouse from Bali and tilt my head in befuddlement. "And, for your information, this is called an empire waist dress, not a maternity gown. I'm not pregnant."

The clerk issues a profusion of apologies and explains that he thought he had seen me walk in holding the hand of a little boy, and thought that I was the mother.

Holy mackerel! I slam the essential oil back on the counter and begin to interrogate the poor man: "What did he look like?"

Likely intimidated by the change in my demeanor, the scrawny clerk replies sheepishly that the child had big round eyes and looked extremely adorable. Holy cow! I take a deep breath.

"Where is he now?" I ask.

"I don't know—the second time you came around he was gone."

"Where do you think he went?"

"Uh—maybe you left him with the maid," he replies, tongue-in-cheek. (Thank you, thank you for not only envisioning me with a child, but also seeing me as a socialite with a maid.)

I ask him, "Do you see things?"

He returns a look of bewilderment.

I lower my voice, "What I mean is, do you occasionally have visions of things that other people cannot see?" He hesitates momentarily, then looks at me and nods.

As a sign of appreciation for this dialog on spirits and the occult so early in the day, I purchase a variety of essential oils with different potencies and uses. As I pay for my goods, the fatigue of travel starts to set in. I head for the powder room with my luggage and shopping bags. After rinsing my face, I survey my appearance in the mirror and use a tissue to wipe away the remaining moisture. I press on the dark circles around my eyes and force a smile, and, as if gazing at an invisible life-form and sharing in a secret yet to be revealed, I say to the baby deep in my heart, "You know, my dear, Mommy has just come back from a faraway place, and she feels as if she is getting ever closer to you."

* From Marula Liu 劉梓潔, *Qinaide xiaohai* 《親愛的小孩》 (*Baby, My Dear*) (Taipei: Crown Publishing, 2013).

CHAPTER 7

NO TIME TO GROW UP

來不及長大

Su Wei-chen 蘇偉貞

(Translated by Patrick Carr 柯英華)

Not even ten years passed between her entering this world and leaving it. Can we really say that she had lived? Who can tell?

The hospital was full of hustle and bustle. The afternoon sun slanted in through the windows between one tall building and another, but it couldn't change anything. The children's ward had an unearthly quiet about it as if glass walls separated it from the world outside, even from time itself.

I wondered if time really had stood still there. Every time I went to see her, there would be a sick child on a tricycle trundling up and down the quiet corridors. The corridors seemed to stretch on forever, like an aimless life. In some of the beds were one- and two-year-old tots, barely able to talk yet already on the verge of death. How much of this world could they understand? Would they remember anything at all? The rows of beds, which constantly changed owners, provided evidence that there wouldn't be time to grow up.

The first time I went to see her I got lost. I never thought the children's ward would be buried so deep within the building, nor that it would be so quiet. It seemed that death was around every corner, waiting quietly to catch me off-guard. Yet I immediately picked her out as she shyly called out to me, "Auntie!" She was most taken with the seaweed snacks that I had brought along and gobbled up piece after piece. She still had the appetite of a child. She was at the twilight of her life.

The corridor was even less lively in the afternoons. A solitary little boy would painstakingly pedal his tricycle down it, stopping to peer in at each doorway to see if any of his friends were still awake. His mother stood just behind him as he looked from room to room, until he got to the end and turned to come back. If the other children weren't lying in bed, disinterested in everything that was going on around them, then they'd been sent home and weren't likely to come back. His thin, pale face didn't show any trace of illness but the doctor said that he had been in and out of the hospital three times already. They feared that this time he might not make it out again.

We would stand at the end of the corridor watching the other children and discussing their illnesses. Everyone knew all the medical details of any given child and how long each of them had left. When it came to her, however, we maintained a kind of blind hope, as if leukemia were a curable disease. As if it surely wouldn't be long until she'd be allowed to go home. Her condition not deteriorating was considered a small victory; everyone's greatest fear was having to come back into the hospital again, and for this reason she was never let outside in bad weather, wasn't allowed to get over-tired, catch a cold, or injure herself. Any small illness or mishap could lead to complications with potentially fatal consequences. After she'd been allowed to go home she had to go back in every week for injections and check-ups. This was something the child found almost impossible to bear; her parents too.

We could hear the noisy afternoon rush-hour traffic, but in the hospital all sounds from outside took on a thin frailty. I never for a moment thought that this was the best it would get. She would only get worse and worse from now on. Her mother related the latest details of her illness in a monotone voice as though directly reporting something someone else had said—but, having recounted the news so many times to so many relatives, how could she be any different?

It had started a year before. She became feverish every now and then, and the doctor had given her injections to ease her temperature. Nevertheless the fevers became increasingly regular until they were more or less constant. Her father was involved in an engineering project overseas and so it was left to her mother to drag her off to the hospital to conduct all sorts of tests. Only when blood bubbles began to appear on her skin did they confirm it as leukemia. What can a child know of leukemia?

Every week they would go to the hospital and every day she would have more injections, more skin and bone marrow samples taken. It was no wonder she hated the hospital. She wanted to eat ice cream, go out and enjoy the sunshine, play with her friends. All of these activities were forbidden. Her parents wanted to preserve her life, to steal any precious time they could from death. Slowly parents and daughter became enemies; that period of her illness was a constant struggle between them.

After she moved into the hospital she began to behave very oddly. The doctor said that one of the side effects of the drugs she was taking was that they caused intense mood swings. She had always been a beautiful child and was most concerned about keeping her good looks. She had taken all of her favorite toys to the hospital and constantly nagged her mother to get her friends to come and see her. Anything that made her happy was a blessing. She was never without her towel, which she would fold and stroke with her hand. Even when the towel became old and smelly she insisted on keeping it as part of a habit carried over from when she was very small. She gained comfort from things that were familiar to her.

Her pretty face and body changed from day to day. One day her eyes would become bloodshot; another she would develop blood bubbles on her tongue. She became unusually weak. She always wanted to be out of the hospital by Saturday because her friends had been watching a TV soap opera from Hong Kong, which they would all be talking about come Monday at school. She had forgotten that it had already been three months since she had last been in class. She had been particularly keen on a boy in another class at school and had proclaimed he was "very handsome and dashing"; but she fretted that she hadn't seen him for so long that he would almost certainly like someone else by now—we teased her by saying we were sure he hadn't forgotten her. How young she was! Before she could start talking seriously about love there were so many things for her to experience. Even this fledgling romance was doomed.

Her mother called me one day to ask whether I could recommend a good fortune-teller and hurried off full of hope to get a reading. She wanted to find a set date amongst all this uncertainty so that she could be sure of at least something; something science couldn't tell her. She hoped that her daughter might have at least a little time left. It was impossible for her to understand how her little one could contract such a terrible illness. There were some who got it even younger.

It wasn't long before the little boy with the tricycle died. The night before, his parents had taken him down south to get a Chinese medicine prescription, returning with a large bag of herbal remedies. They boiled up the roots using a small gas stove right there in the ward as he pedaled down the corridor as usual, looking into each room as he went. The medicine was bitter. He was only four when he passed away.

The trundling sound of the tricycle didn't go away though. Any illness that adults can contract, children can get too, and nothing can prepare you for the vice-like grip of a debilitating disease.

She had questions for the doctor: "What is leukemia? Is it the sort of disease that makes people very ugly?" She asked her mother, too: "Am I going to die? If it hurts this much, wouldn't it be better to die a little sooner anyway?" Her mother replied that then she would leave her little sister all on her own. She said that if she died earlier she could be reincarnated and her mother could have another child. She would remember the way back home in her new body and maybe she would be reincarnated as a boy to keep dad company! Her sister might even become a bit more "girly" in the bargain. She said, "Wouldn't it be better like that?" Her mother asked what would happen if she couldn't remember the way home? She resolved to continue enduring her illness and live a little longer.

As long as she continued to breathe each day, her parents could never bear to let her go; but what was the point of living on like that? If only she didn't open her eyes again it would all be over.

As she began to lose her hair, they had to hide all the mirrors. At first it came out a few strands at a time, then in great handfuls, but there was no way of stopping it. Someone moved into the next-door bed. There were always more relatives visiting at the beginning. They would exchange the latest news of illness in the corridors; it was like looking at ourselves in the past. From their faces you could detect a mixture of shock, sorrow, and hope. They were still optimistic that it mightn't be too long before he would get out of the hospital. If he were lucky maybe he could steal forty or fifty years in spite of the time bomb he carried inside him; by then all manner of medical miracles might be possible and such illnesses would be a thing of the past. We didn't have to ask what illness their child was suffering from; just seeing the flow of relatives come and go was enough. If they didn't see him now it would be too late.

Her hair covered the bed and pillow whenever she laid down for long. Jet black yet dull and lifeless, she couldn't bear to cut it, yet it fell out of its own accord. Her fluffy long hair piled around her head like a bird's nest while her mother helped her comb it. When great clumps come out she left them where they were, reluctant to take away so much at a time. She held her hair, crying as she did so but at the same time wanting a mirror. It had been a long time since she had last looked in a mirror. She refused to let her friends come and see her because she felt she looked so ugly and pleaded with her mother to buy her a wig—a short-haired one would do fine; long hair would only fall out and there was no point in having it so long anyway.

She got thinner and thinner. Only her arms and legs remained beautiful. Her young buck teeth jutted out from her angular face and looked depressing precisely because of their conspicuousness. She received injections and transfusions almost every day. Whenever she felt a little better she would ask when her dad was coming home. He finally returned. On the plane home he couldn't help himself from weeping when he saw the air hostesses; she used to say that when she grew up she wanted to be an air hostess so she could take her dad around the world. The moment she was born her father had clapped his hands together and exclaimed, "What a wonder!" and the nickname had stuck. The two of them forged a strong bond; they were thick as thieves and kept all sorts of secrets between them. Her father made plans, including for when he would become a grandfather—it was Wonder who made him truly understand what it was to be a father. They had met each other in a hospital, and now they met there again. Matters of life and death are beyond the control even of parents. Is everything indeed predestined? In spite of the intricacy and precision of science and technology, there is simply no answer to this riddle.

A small bed was made up next to hers where her father kept vigil night and day, day after day. The bed was too short for his six-foot frame, so he slept with most of his body hanging off the end. Illness is excruciatingly tedious; he would help pass the time by telling her stories, all of which she had heard a dozen times before. The city could not supply her with new material fast enough; she had read every fairytale, every comic, and seen every cartoon. She became bored and took to stroking her towel more and more frequently. Each time I went to see her now she would be stroking it, changing hands when she got tired. The hospital had a teacher who could give private tutorials once a week; he could even bring exam papers in for her to complete, but she soon lost interest. At the beginning she worried that she wouldn't be able to keep up with her classmates, but she was a bright girl and always got good grades. Eventually she gave it up completely. After all, she didn't have any classmates; who could she compare herself against?

Other kids grew up out in the sunshine. One day she told her father, "I don't even remember what the sun feels like!" Those other children had probably forgotten they ever had such a classmate.

Although the hospital was quiet, it was far too quiet. Every second felt like a final breath. People here lived their lives on tiptoe, afraid that they would disturb others. The atmosphere in rooms with older patients seemed louder and less inhibited. However desperate their plight now, they could at least have said that they had had lived some kind of life. It was only in the children's wards that one could be shocked by each and every one of the kids lying prone in their beds. We are so used to thinking of them as indestructible. Because they haven't grown up yet, we don't tend to think of them as people, more almost as small "life vessels." Can death really be serious about invading such a potent force? And how can it possibly have inveigled its way in? We made believe that one day she would grow up tall and strong and be transformed into a young lady, but her body simply vanished before it took any definite form, as if what had died was just the soul. It made my heart bleed to see her like this, especially once her illness could get neither better nor worse.

In the neighboring room there was a baby that was entirely cocooned in an incubator; too young even to be able to call out for his mother; his mother couldn't even hold him in her arms.

Rather than waste her last months trapped in the hospital they decided to take her home. They wanted the normality of all four of them being back under one roof. If they were careful she might not get worse and they could spend some time together as a family. Their youngest daughter had been overlooked for far too long.

They bought Wonder a wig and took a whole stack of photos. She smiled silently out from the pictures, her likeness suspended forever in another space and time, missing from her relatives' and friends' get-togethers. In reaction to the side effects of the drugs she was taking, her body began to swell up. Her normally thin face blew up as if filled with air, making her look entirely different. She no longer wanted to look in the mirror for fear of not recognizing her own reflection; she told her mother she would wait till she got better before looking again. Her mother took up religion and gained faith from the Psalms, hoping that by willpower alone she could change her daughter's fate. Her father had to go abroad again to carry out a contract he had already signed—but what about the contract from birth between father and daughter? He asked her to wait until he returned. She contracted an infection and developed painfully itchy sores all around her waist, known as "dragons girdling the waist," which meant that she couldn't take any medicine or have injections. Her father went abroad as she was readmitted into the hospital.

There were a few new children in the hospital and the bed Wonder had been in was occupied, so she was moved to a different room along the corridor. Her mother gave up her job to stay at her bedside night and day. Her younger daughter was packed off to stay with relatives. It was almost as if her daughter's illness was the thing that kept her going day after day. People's reports of her condition got worse and worse. The doctors said it looked as though she had simply given up.

The next time I went to see her I couldn't remember the ward and got lost again. The atmosphere in the hospital was the same as usual. The little boy who loved to ride his tricycle was nowhere to be seen on the long corridor, and it was even quieter than before. I stood outside a room and saw a little girl of around three facing me through the window. She had a beautifully pale, delicate face and the old woman caring for her played with her so that she seemed the happiest child in the world. She rocked her head to and fro, swinging the sparse hair on her head. For a second it looked not as though her hair had fallen out, but as if it hadn't grown yet; the aged young face made a startling picture. I stood rooted to the spot in the doorway. I had found the right room, but the little girl in the bed was a total stranger. I barely even recognized the woman sitting with her back to me. She quickly turned around; her nerves meant that even the slightest disturbance made her flinch. Her face was haggard. A whole year of distress had turned her into an old woman. She got up and said to Wonder, "Auntie's here to see you!"

Wonder kept both eyes tightly shut, as if she hadn't heard. Her mother said that she was too tired even to open her eyes, not to mention saying anything. They asked her why she always shook her head, lying still day and night, refusing to give even a small clue as to the thoughts in her head. What in heaven's name was she thinking? No one could tell. Her mother cajoled her into looking at the cartoon sweets Auntie had brought her; each and every cartoon character on the candy jar was smiling a broad grin. She opened her eyes but could only manage a weak, unfocused glance, a gaze so shockingly empty of expression it made the heart miss a beat. How could a child possess such a look?

The girl in the bed next to hers was still laughing, facing the window, oblivious of us at her back. Her mother started telling me the latest news. Death wasn't even mentioned in passing, yet its shadow was everywhere, thickening the air, smothering the child.

Since she had been back in the hospital, every second seemed like borrowed time. People often feel time passing, but to literally see time fly by is terrifying. Against this overwhelming pressure she had no power to resist. All her mother could do was be there for her little girl.

All her hair fell out but she only wore her wig for a short time; she never went out, had no mirrors to look at herself in, and could barely even open her eyes let alone think about what she looked like to others. A few wisps of hair appeared on her swollen head, as if they were the first hairs on a baby's head, but her frail body had stopped growing altogether. She kept her beautifully slender arms crossed feebly over her chest. When I would later think back on it, those beautiful arms are the only thing I can remember clearly. Disease is heartless. Brutal. She was once such a beautiful girl.

As I walked past the line of rooms, looking in at each face, I realized I would never run into any of them again by chance at some point in the future. Maybe one or two, but not many. Leaving the children's ward, I ran into a mass of bustling humanity. In times of sickness grown-ups seem to be so much more outwardly expressive. I have seen people dying of cancer shouting and weeping, cursing and wailing. Why is it, then, that children pass away with such little fuss? Is it that they don't know the difference between life and death, or that they simply resist in silence?

It was early morning when she died.

She opened her eyes and weakly called out to her grandmother sitting beside her, "I need to poo." Her grandmother pulled aside the covers and changed her nappy; it was full of blood. She closed her eyes again and looked as if even breathing was too much of an effort for her. Her grandmother cleaned her up and called a nurse to change the sheets. After they tucked her in she opened her eyes again and said again, "I need to poo." Having pulled off the covers and taken off her nappy, once again soaked in blood, her grandmother sprinkled talcum powder over her as if looking after a newborn baby with no control over its bowel movements. She tried to speak, but hadn't the strength to make a sound.

Her parents hurried straight to the hospital, and her little sister was sent for. Her grandmother said, "Wonder, your sister's here; why don't you say hi to her?" She shook her head. Her grandmother asked her to open her eyes so she could get a good look at them all. She briefly opened her eyes but closed them again without appearing to have registered anything. Her mother said, "Wonder, look at Mummy; remember Mummy's face so you can find your way back safely!" She stretched out her hand for the pen to write with, but couldn't hold it steady and gave up with a sigh, closing her eyes again. Her grandmother said, "Wonder, do you want to go now?" She nodded her head. "Does it hurt a lot?" She nodded again.

Her grandmother rested the tips of her fingers on her eyelids and said, "You just go, then." She nodded again.

Her parents arranged a Requiem Mass for her. There was no weeping and wailing; they knew that over the last year every day had only brought her more pain and suffering. She would always live on for them as their ten-year-old girl. Even if every family in the rest of the world seemed to have two children, they didn't want another.

Children don't know the difference between life and death, but death comes and claims them anyway.

* From *Tien-hsia san-wen hsuan* er 《天下散文選 II》 (*CommonWealth's Selection of Essays, Vol. II*), eds. Choong Yee Voon 鍾怡雯 and Chen Ta-wei 陳大為 (Taipei: CommonWealth, 2001).

CHAPTER 8

A PLACE OF ONE'S OWN

自己的天空

Yuan Chiung-chiung 袁瓊瓊

(Translated by Jane Parish Yang 白珍)

She suddenly began to cry.

Lips pressed tightly shut, Liang-san[1] sat there before her in silence and said nothing more. Tears streamed down her face as she looked at him, and her cheeks burned. She didn't know why, but all she could think about was that burning, itching sensation. She didn't know how Liang-san felt facing a crying woman, or how Liang-ssu and Liang-ch'i felt. The three large men sat around the table watching her cry. Tears blurred her vision. All she saw before her were three heads held high, but she couldn't make out their expressions.

"Sister-in-law," Liang-ch'i said. The blur in his direction moved. Ching-min looked down and tried to find her handkerchief in her purse. She heard Liang-ch'i repeat "Sister-in-law" as she dried her eyes.

"Uh..." she answered. Her vision cleared. Liang-san and Liang-ssu both looked down to avoid her eyes, their faces expressionless. Liang-ch'i was still a youth and unable to control his feelings. He sat there red-faced.

Ching-min looked at him and he suddenly stood up. "Why'd you make me come here anyway?" His voice broke.

Liang-ssu tugged at him. "Sit down."

Liang-ch'i sat down. Ching-min saw his eyes were red. When she was first married, he had still been in elementary school. Up until he entered high school, he had gotten along best with her, his sister-in-law. Now it seemed that he was the only one sympathetic to her. Heart-broken, she began to cry again.

"Didn't you already agree that you wouldn't cry?" Liang-san said slowly. He paused, then continued speaking in the tone of a superior to an inferior. "This isn't home, you know."

Ching-min wiped her eyes.

Liang-ssu played the role of mediator between them. He chimed in, "Don't cry, Sister-in-law. Liang-san didn't say he didn't want you."

Liang-san said, "That's right." He spoke without a trace of shame. "It's only a temporary arrangement. She's making a big fuss right now. It's just a cover-up to calm her down." "She" referred to that dancing girl.

When he mentioned that woman, a faint smile crept over his face, but just for an instant. Ching-min saw it clearly but couldn't understand how he could be so heartless. After all, they had been husband and wife for seven years. If other men had mistresses, their wives would have raised the roof. Only he could have arranged everything so neatly. He didn't take her seriously at all. And now he even wanted her to move out so that other woman could move in. He took it for granted that she'd obey.

Liang-ssu said, "The apartment Liang-san's rented for you is an efficiency. It's a little small, but it's got everything."

Liang-san said, "It's a nice place to stay." He frowned, but not out of vexation. It was an expression of solemnity and resolution. "I'll go visit you every week."

Silence. Ching-min wiped her eyes with her handkerchief. The slight rustling sound blended with her breathing. She inhaled and exhaled heavily, as if having caught a cold.

Liang-ch'i folded his arms in front of his body and stared at her gloomily, as if he had suddenly turned into her enemy. Liang-ssu was the slickest operator in the family, and now his face was arranged in a solemn expression. Liang-san's face was a blank, as if he were about to doze off. He rarely looked so friendly. Perhaps he, too, had a conscience and felt he might be going a bit too far.

Ching-min finally spoke up. "Why?"

The three men stared at her. She fell silent, bowing her head to think. Strangely, she discovered her mind was a blank.

This was an important matter for a woman. Her husband was having an affair and now wanted to separate. But she couldn't think of anything else, not even of crying. Then why had she just cried? Maybe because she had always cried easily, or because she had been taken by surprise. She hadn't thought this kind of thing could happen to her. Perhaps it was because she felt unhappy that they hadn't talked it over at home, but that he had brought her here, the four of them sitting around a large round table like they were waiting to be served. It was absurd. By coincidence all the booths were full so the brothers sat at one side of the table and she sat alone across from them as if they had nothing to do with each other.

She ought to have given a more appropriate response, such as rebuking Liang-san's ingratitude. *What have I done wrong that you'd treat me this way?* There was a lot of that shown on television. *The least I should do is faint*, she thought. But she merely sat there, painlessly healthy, her hands gripping her handkerchief under the table. She crumbled it up, then released it. She noticed a cigarette burn in the carpet. The carpet was deep red with a black pattern. Unless one looked closely, the hole didn't show. She wiped her face with the handkerchief again, guessing that her face looked terrible. She was afraid her nose was all puffy. She suddenly felt ashamed to appear this ugly at the time he wanted to leave her.

Liang-san said, "She'll give birth in June. She needs a bigger place."

Ching-min became despondent. She replied, "Oh." She felt stricken when he mentioned the child. She and Liang-san didn't have any children, but she hadn't known he wanted a child so badly. He had never said anything about it. She suddenly felt like crying again and the tears came flowing down her cheeks. The men were silent. She clearly saw a tear drop onto her skirt, the sound seeming horribly loud, like rain beating on the pavement.

The door to the elegant private dining room opened. The waiter had finally shown up. The restaurant was very busy. Ching-min sat with her head bowed.

Liang-san said, "Let's eat something! This place is famous." He looked over the menu quietly, calmly soliciting the others' opinions. "How about an order of shrimp balls?"

The waiter scribbled it down on his notepad.

Liang-ssu said, "Let's order something a little less rich. Liang-san, this won't do. You'd better be careful about high blood pressure."

"This dish is their specialty, understand?" Liang-san ordered four dishes and a soup.

The waiter departed.

"I think I'll go to the ladies' room," Ching-min said, her head still bowed.

"Go on then," Liang-san said.

Getting up, Ching-min fumbled in her purse for something, then finally decided to take it along. The three men sat there politely in silence. Liang-ssu even smiled faintly.

Ching-min closed the door. On the other side was the family of three brothers who called her wife and sister-in-law. But at this moment she was shut out and felt at a loss for what to do. She just stood there in a daze. Warm, pungent fragrances from the restaurant kitchen came floating over to her as she walked along the hall. At the end was the kitchen, where she could see the chef's white hat and apron and the stainless steel cabinets. Around the corner was the restaurant and beyond the many tables and chairs crowded with people was the automatic door. It was of brown glass, which made the outside seem dark like evening. Ching-min looked, wanting to walk right out. The hum of voices buzzed in her ears. But if she left, what would she do next? She felt frustrated. For all seven years of her marriage she had always depended on Liang-san. She'd never even gone out alone on her own. She didn't even know where this place was. Besides, she hadn't brought much money because she was always with him. And now he had brought her here to tell her this. She had believed in him, but he didn't take her seriously at all.

She was angry at herself for not being more competent. Why hadn't she even brought some money? There were too many things she wasn't up to doing. Before, when she went out, it had always been Liang-san who picked her up and took her home. She doubted whether she could even direct a taxi in the right direction. She was really incompetent. No wonder he wanted to get rid of her. To him it was just as easy as throwing out an old newspaper.

All she could do was head for the ladies' room. She looked in the mirror and saw that in fact her face was a mess. She washed her face and looked in the mirror to put on her make-up. After crying, her eyes sparkled. She looked closely at her reflection in the mirror, feeling she looked quite spirited, not like a woman who had just received a crushing blow. But why take this as a crushing blow anyway? She didn't feel she loved Liang-san that much. They had been introduced to each other by a match-maker. It was a quiet marriage that hadn't required any effort.

Perhaps Liang-san felt more deeply toward that other woman. When he mentioned her, his whole expression changed.

But she had cried so much just now. Liang-san probably thought she'd had a mental breakdown. His whole idea had been to first shock her, then pacify her. He didn't want her to entangle herself around him and make a fool of herself. He didn't know she didn't care one way or the other. She had kept on crying because she was scared. Besides, she remembered she was almost thirty years old and was suddenly an outcast woman. If this had happened several years earlier, she would still have been considered young. She couldn't quite think how being a bit younger when cast out was an advantage, but everything seemed better when one was young. She began to hate Liang-san, as if he had dumped a bucket of cold water over her as she lay soaking in a hot bath. She began to make her face up very carefully. It was for Liang-san. She had always made herself up on account of him. But, having just put her eyeliner on, she wiped it off again. This, too, was on account of Liang-san. If she looked too stunning, he'd probably feel unhappy. He had always thought that he was everything to her.

When she returned to the private dining room, the three had already begun to eat. Liang-san looked up at her and said, "How about eating a little something!"

This was just like at home, the family sitting around and eating. Liang-ch'i didn't look at her at all. Ching-min didn't know why, but she sensed a strong sense of shame in him, as if he were the only one here in the family who had done something wrong. She knew he sympathized with her. Maybe Liang-ssu did, too, but he didn't have such a strong moral sense. He picked out a lotus-leaf-wrapped steamed meat and gingerly spread the leaf apart with his chopsticks. Liang-san was always in a good mood when he ate. He slowly related how he had discovered this restaurant and directed Ching-min's attention to the dishes as he always had done in the past. "Ching-min, you should study how they did this. They really know how to cook here."

Liang-ssu asked, "She's not very good at things like that, is she?" He didn't look at Ching-min. He wasn't referring to her. "...with her background."

Liang-san looked a bit regretful. "That's true!"

Ching-min sat in silence, a bit unhappy that they would talk about that woman right in front of her like this.

Liang-san seemed to want to pacify her. "Ching-min really is a good cook. That's really hard to find."

His praise for her was probably limited to just these words. Liang-san was a real connoisseur. Actually, all the men in his family were. She sympathized with him at the thought that the new woman of his didn't know how to cook. In that instant she thought of him as just another man and sympathized with him that his wife was no good. She forgot he was her own husband.

Ching-min said, "Too bad you won't get to taste it anymore."

Liang-san laid his chopsticks down and looked at her. "What?"

"My cooking!" Ching-min replied slowly. She suddenly felt a sense of release. "I don't want to separate."

Liang-san looked up and blanched. "Didn't we just agree to it?"

"Let's get a divorce."

Ching-min felt a sense of satisfaction when the three brothers all stared at her at once. Their expressions differed, though. Besides, Liang-ch'i was thin and Liang-san had a round face. But all the men in the family looked a lot alike.

This was how Ching-min got divorced. When she told people, they reprimanded her: "How could you have been so stupid?"

Liu Fen reprimanded her as well. "How could anybody be so foolish? Why'd you lay it out so clearly? No one will even sympathize with you."

Liu Fen was two years younger than she was and a divorcée as well. Hers was another kind of marriage. She had gotten pregnant in high school. Forced to get married, she never adjusted to married life and so had gotten a divorce. Before she turned twenty all the important events in a woman's life had already happened to her. Her mother raised the child. She took good care of herself, not looking at all as if she'd had a child already. She saw her former husband often, too. She said, "As long as he's not my husband, I think he's really adorable."

Ching-min used the money Liang-san gave her when they divorced to open a handicraft shop. It was small and she didn't hire any help so usually had more business than she could attend to. Liu Fen would come over at those times to help out. She was a seamstress in a shop across the street. When not busy, she liked to go over and chat with Ching-min. The two would sit on the step in front of the store like grade-school kids. In the afternoon when there was a breeze, it was a cool spot.

Liu Fen was used to plopping right down and crossing her legs. When it was hot out, she'd even wear shorts. She leaned over and patted Ching-min. "How come you're so ladylike? At first I thought you were some cultured lady!"

Ching-min sat with her legs together and feet tucked under her. She was used to sitting in a constrained manner and couldn't loosen up all at once.

Liu Fen looked absently toward the entrance to the lane. Her son would be getting out of school soon. He was in fourth grade and already really tall and sturdy. Liu Fen went on chatting about the news in the paper about Ts'ui T'ai-ch'ing. "They're already divorced so why hate him so much? As soon as Hsiao-ping and I were divorced I didn't hate him anymore. We weren't fighting or hitting each other anymore."

Hsiao-ping was only a year older than she was. They both had fiery tempers. They were no longer husband and wife, but when Hsiao-ping came to stay overnight they'd still quarrel with each other upstairs. The next day the garbage pail would be full of broken objects. "Hsiao-ping is coming today," she said slowly, thinking of something.

"Really?" Ching-min replied. "You haven't been fighting much lately."

"Eh?" Liu Fen said, startled. "That's not fighting. You don't know what it was like before. It was as if I were a guy. He'd beat me up!" She concluded, "Hsiao-ping has matured a lot."

Someone came into the lane. Liu Fen had sharp eyes. "Hey, Little Hsieh's here again." She mocked Liang-ch'i by calling him "Little Hsieh." She raised her voice listlessly from the step in front of the store. "Hey, Little Hsieh!"

Liang-ch'i came over to them, his face rigid. Liu Fen didn't pay any attention. She grabbed him and made him sit down on the step. "You haven't been here for a long time."

Liang-ch'i looked past Liu Fen to greet Ching-min. "Sister Ching-min." She had forgotten when he had begun calling her "Sister Ching-min."

Ching-min replied, "I'll get you a glass of cold water."

She brought out two glasses of cold water. She looked at Liang-ch'i from behind. He had lost weight. His shirt hung on him.

She sat down and asked, "How come you've lost so much weight?"

Liu Fen answered for him, "He's been taking tests and staying up late."

She finished off the cold water and went back to her store.

Ching-min sat on the steps with Liang-ch'i. Between them was the empty space where Liu Fen had been sitting. She had a funny feeling when the wind blew. It was as if they were sitting so close but there was still a distance between them.

Liang-ch'i often came to see her. He was the only one in the Hsieh family to feel bad. He always had something on his mind. He sounded like he was angry with himself. "It's the baby's one-month anniversary."

Liang-san had had a daughter. Liang-ch'i looked down at his feet. "Liang-san wanted a son."

"Oh," Ching-min answered gently. "Men are always like that."

Liang-ch'i protested, "I'm not." He looked away from her as he spoke.

"Well, it's too early for you anyway." Ching-min smiled at him. She looked over at the back of his head. His hair was always too long, thick and disheveled. She reached over as she spoke and tugged at his hair. "Your hair's really long."

Liang-ch'i was startled and replied recklessly, "Who's to cut it for me?"

"Let me do it, alright? I'm not bad with my hands." She had learned how from a magazine, but she had actually done it only on Liu Fen and herself. She turned her head to show Liang-ch'i. "Look at my hair. I did it myself."

Liang-ch'i turned around and stared at her awkwardly, his eyes soft and liquid. Ching-min couldn't help flirting with him. She leaned closer. "Well, how about it?" She felt astonished when she blurted it out. Liang-ch'i had always been a younger brother-in-law to her. She had watched him grow up. But just then she had treated him like any ordinary man.

She looked around for a sheet and wrapped him up in it. He didn't like the heat so she placed an electric fan in front of him. She first dampened his hair with a spray bottle. His wet hair plastered against his skull made his head look a lot smaller. Liang-ch'i sat there obediently, his whole body encased in the sheet, only his head sticking out for her to work on. Ching-min first pinned his hair up and said to him, "You look like a co-ed." She smiled down at him. Liang-ch'i looked up at her without moving his head.

She said, "Do you remember I used to wash your hair for you when you were little?"

Liang-ch'i said, "Yes." She didn't know why he answered so formally; Ching-min felt like laughing. When she'd had contact with him before, he had been a mischievous little boy. Now he was really grown up. He hadn't even shaved his mustache, probably because he'd been busy with finals. A visible dark streak lined his upper lip. Young men's skins were smooth and looked so clean. Liang-ch'i sat with his lips pursed. He always looked like that.

The hair she cut off smelled of tobacco smoke. Ching-min sighed, "How long has it been since you washed your hair?"

Liang-ch'i replied, "No one to wash it for me!"

"How about your own hands?"

"You've got them tied up." He moved his hands under the sheet.

They were silent for a moment, then Ching-min said, "Well, I'm not going to do it for you." She added, "Lazy."

School had just let out and the lane gradually filled with students. Some came to buy thread. Some girls crowded around the counter. Ching-min went over to wait on them. Her business was always like this. It came in spurts. The girls knew her well. They burst out laughing. "Mistress, you can cut hair?"

Liang-ch'i sat stonily on the counter, the clips still in his hair. He shut his eyes as if angry. He was probably embarrassed. Ching-min ordered him, "Liang-ch'i, go sit inside." Inside was her bedroom. Liang-ch'i went inside the back room. She explained to the others, "My little brother." She turned to another girl and said, "That's my younger brother." Actually, no one paid any attention to what she was saying. She taught several of them some embroidery stiches. She took out the colors and background with printed borders to show them. She finally finished waiting on them and hurriedly went into the back room. The store and back room were only separated by a curtain. She pushed it aside and went in, calling out, "Liang-ch'i."

He had already taken off the sheet. He was sitting on the bed leafing through the weekly TV listings. The curtain clacked together behind her. She had made it herself out of wooden beads. Shards of the world outside were visible between the beads.

In the room was a vanity table, a single bed, and a chair, with cardboard boxes and other materials in the corner. With Liang-ch'i in the room, she suddenly felt it had gotten a lot smaller. She stood awkwardly with her back against the curtain. "Liang-ch'i, are you angry?"

"No." He put the magazine down. "Sister Ching-min, you've changed. You're so capable." He gestured and added mischievously, "I don't mean you weren't capable before, though."

"Let me cut your hair again."

This time she had him sit in front of the vanity table. After cutting for a while, she discovered that Liang-ch'i was watching her in the mirror. She stopped and asked, "What's the matter?"

"What do you mean what's the matter?"

"You keep staring at me." She made a face like a shrew. She had watched him grow up. She wasn't embarrassed in front of him.

He said, "Then who should I watch?"

"Look at yourself!"

Liang-ch'i replied, "Alright," and the two burst into laughter. Ching-min asked cautiously, "Do you have a girlfriend?"

"Not yet." He even pursed his lips when he laughed, and looked even more mischievous. Ching-min looked at him in the mirror and suddenly felt a bit shaky. Perhaps Liang-ch'i's clean-cut features seemed especially bright in the mirror's reflection. His face narrowed to his chin, its smooth outline very handsome. The clumps of hair in her hand were wet and glossy as silk. She felt as if she couldn't stop herself from sinking into his arms. Her head felt heavy. Body odor from Liang-ch'i floated up toward her, the faint smell of cigarette smoke and perspiration. She had never had a male in this room before.

Ching-min was afraid of herself.

She said, "I'm going to watch the store a minute." She lifted the curtain and went out.

Liang-ch'i followed her, taking the sheet off as he went. The hair clips were still in his hair. Ching-min felt like laughing. She lifted the curtain up and went back inside. Liang-ch'i followed again.

He suddenly spoke up. "Sister Ching-min. I really like you." He stood with his back to the curtain, the world shut away beyond him. In his crazy, damp unfinished hair, the gray hair clips rested on his head like giant moths. He was scared, too, and, having spoken, pursed his lips tightly as he stood there. He was a grown-up but his slender frail frame seemed to invite one to embrace him like a child.

Perhaps he had been thinking about this too long. Once having spoken up, he was like a taut string that suddenly snapped. He wasn't smiling. His expression was determined.

They didn't know what to do. They just stood there. At last Ching-min said, "Come over and let me finish cutting your hair." Liang-ch'i went over and sat quietly in front of the mirror.

She began to cry. She'd probably never be able to change this part of her. Liang-ch'i tried to get up but she pushed him down. Tears fell onto his hair as she proceeded to cut it. She wiped the tears away as she cut. Liang-ch'i anxiously apologized, "Sister Ching-min, I'm sorry."

"Never mind. I just like to cry." Liang-ch'i was dumbstruck. Ching-min sensed the fearsomeness in herself. She wasn't weeping hysterically, just sobbing silently, her eyes welling with tears as if she were finding release from daily injustices. Actually, that wasn't true. Having left Liang-san, she felt she had gotten along quite well on her own. Men just weren't that important. Whenever she was in a foul mood she'd cry. She'd cry when she read novels or watched movies on TV, too. Thinking of this, she laughed again and Liang-ch'i, watching her in the mirror, was reassured. He smiled back sheepishly.

Ching-min said, "It's just that I like to cry. It has nothing to do with you."

She cut his hair with care. She did like Liang-ch'i somewhat, but not to that degree. He was still young; just look at the way he'd stopped worrying right away. She was angry with herself. She had been divorced less than a year but still cried when a man said he liked her!

"Liang-ch'i, that's nonsense," Ching-min said, but sensed her tone wasn't quite right. She took the scissors and rapped him on the head: "I'm your Third Sister-in-law!"

Having finished cutting his hair, she washed it for him. The two squeezed into the narrow little bathroom. Liang-ch'i bent over and lowered his head into the sink. Ching-min reached over and gripped his head with her left hand. A man this intimate with her was like a younger brother, lover, or son.

The cool water splashed out of the faucet and flowed over her fingers. Between her fingers were his long locks, like small black snakes curled on the back of her hand. The hair in the water floated up like strands of silk, in an orderly and beautiful fashion. She'd probably remember this for the rest of her life. In the afternoon there wasn't a sound outside. The old electric fan buzzed noisily in the front room, spluttering from right to left as it turned, then back again. The apartment was not new and the bathroom smelled mildewed. The fragrant scent of the shampoo seemed to cover the mildew smell as well as the acrid perspiration from Liang-ch'i. He lowered his head to let the water wet his hair. The parts she touched were all cool. He was quiet and obedient but breathed heavily. She knew he was in an awkward position. She felt the same way. She breathed carefully, inhaling only a little each time, then when she could no longer hold back, she exhaled deeply as if sighing. The two of them were pressed tightly together. Liang-ch'i's breathing came rapidly as if they were committing an indiscretion, but they weren't.

After this she became restless and was always on edge. She finally got rid of the store and began selling policies for an insurance company. This was the only work she could find.

She carried big packets of information wherever she went and greeted people wreathed in smiles. She couldn't believe that she could do this. She wasn't particularly eloquent but she looked sincere. She didn't force the policies on people. She just sat there and spread the information out for them to see, and she read the pertinent portions to prospective customers in a candid manner. Whatever they said she'd only reply slowly with a "Yes..." Her stretching the word out over several seconds made people think she had something to say but didn't dare. Prospective customers found it hard not to sympathize with her. If they turned her down, they would always call her back sometime later. Her sales record was excellent and she began to move up in the organization, becoming a section manager.

She was darker and thinner now. She wore jeans because they were convenient. She wasn't as shy as before. Her eyes sparkled and she had learned to cross her legs up high when she sat down. Her smile was warm and bright without any trace of slyness. When people saw her this way, they let most of their defenses down.

She met Ch'u Shao-chieh when she was out selling insurance. They began living together soon afterward. This time it was she who was the other woman. She knew he was married but she liked that tough-guy appearance of his. A spoiled man over forty, he hadn't yet learned how to live. He was the manager of an import-export company when Ching-min came bursting into his luminous office all of glass, stainless steel, acrylic, plastic, and aluminum. Ch'u Shao-chieh sat behind his desk, clean face and hair, wearing a freshly pressed suit. He listened to her impatiently, his face in a scowl, tough and stubborn-looking. He had insurance. He didn't need to take out any more. He didn't want to discuss it. Sorry. He had other things to take care of.

He was still polite and escorted her to the door. He wore aftershave cologne, the scent of green olives.

Ching-min decided she wanted him. She was thirty-three then, having been out on her own in society for four years. She had begun changing into a confident woman. Besides learning how to dress and make herself up, she had learned how to use people, learned how to deal with different kinds of people and what words were most effective in getting what she wanted. She paid attention to details and was willing to sit quietly and listen to others talk, with the result that she learned how to sympathize with others' feelings and imagine their way of thinking.

She understood what kind of person Ch'u Shao-chieh was.

The second time she went to him, she dressed in a very feminine manner—a thin silk dress, her hair neatly combed close to her face. She only took up ten minutes of his time and didn't talk about insurance.

After that she went there often, and her visits increased in length. Sometimes they went out to eat together. She fell in love with him then, and it was as if her mind was suddenly a blank and she didn't take anything into consideration. All she could think of was him. Her confidence disappeared. She dressed up every day and floated gracefully into his office. She would sit in a dignified manner, her legs tucked underneath the chair, and watch him closely. Her whole person was fluent and elegant. Anyone could tell she was brimming over like a vase filled with water. Anyone except him, that is. He would knit his thick, handsome brows obstinately. He was intractable. Whenever she came he'd raise his eyebrows. "You're back to sell insurance?"

Ching-min couldn't stand it anymore. She became afraid when she discovered she was in love. She couldn't take this kind of seriousness. She loved him so much she felt her whole body was translucent. In front of him, she was as sensitive as a fragile grass that retracted at the slightest touch. She was a grown-up. Wasn't she a little too old to play this game? She stopped going to see him, as if she had forgotten all about him. But she couldn't give him up. She finally went back again and decided to come to terms with this affair. She didn't even know how he felt about her.

Ch'u Shao-chieh hadn't changed a bit, as if all this time he had been nailed to his chair at his office desk without having left once. He looked up and arched his thick black eyebrows. "You're back to sell insurance?"

He hadn't even changed those words.

Ching-min cried once more.

She finally got him to buy some insurance. Shortly afterward, they began living together.

When she told Liu Fen about all of these happenings, it sounded relatively simple. She recounted it in two or three sentences: "I tried to get him to buy insurance but he kept on refusing. I went there every day to pester him." She held Liu Fen's new son in one arm. He was plump and heavy and holding him made her arm ache. She switched arms. Liu Fen reached over, "Let me hold him!"

"And then?"

Ching-min said, "Later we got acquainted, and he finally bought some insurance!"

Liu Fen looked at her and passed judgment: "It looks to me like you're doing okay." She explained, "You really look beautiful."

"Oh," Ching-min giggled.

Liu Fen married Hsiao-ping again. They opened a restaurant in the city with Liu Fen as cashier behind the counter. She had grown heavier. Sitting at the counter, she looked plump and white like a steamed bun just out of the bamboo steamer. She put the baby on the counter and wiped the saliva from his mouth.

Ching-min played with him. "Let's not eat anything but this little piglet!" She nipped at him. "Take a bite. Take a bite."

Some customers entered. The waitresses were busy so Liu Fen went over to wait on them herself. She called out, "Sit over here! What can I bring you?"

Ching-min had become the child's godmother the moment he was born. They got along famously. She wondered if she really could get pregnant or not. Maybe she was just too old. She really wanted a child by Shao-chieh.

Liu Fen came over and patted her on the back. "Ching-min, the people at that table asked about you."

"Which table?" This happened a lot. She had met many people while selling insurance.

"Come with me." Ching-min smiled, picked the child up and squeezed past the other tables. A couple was sitting at a table with two children. The wife stared at her from afar, very cautiously. The man was wiping one of the children's hands, his face to one side. When Ching-min came closer, he finally looked up.

It was Liang-san.

Ching-min called out, "Why it's Liang-san!" She really was a little pleased. Both sides introduced themselves. Liu Fen took the child back with her. Ching-min said enthusiastically, "I haven't seen you in ages!"

All these years of experience had trained her in this kind of greeting. Liang-san looked startled, then smiled and said politely, "You've changed a lot." The two at this moment had no common past. Liang-san seemed like a new acquaintance. Ching-min felt that though she had forgotten many things, she didn't think he had been like this. She couldn't remember what he had been like, though.

She stood holding on to the back of a chair. Their family of four filled the four chairs at the table, and they didn't make any move to let her sit down. Ching-min therefore squeezed onto the seat with the older daughter. This was something she wouldn't have done in the past. She saw Liang-san's strange expression. He repeated, "You've changed a lot!"

"Everyone changes!" She smiled. She had a strange feeling that she had become two different persons. She rarely thought about what she had been like in the past, but facing Liang-san, her former self reappeared. She suddenly and forcefully felt the great change between her past and present self. She smiled, holding her chin lazily in her hand. She knew she was making that woman uneasy.

"Liang-san, you've changed a lot, too!"

"No, I haven't," Liang-san denied hurriedly.

"You're fatter."

"I'm not, either!" He still denied it. He suddenly seemed so pitifully ingenuous.

They chatted a bit about what they were doing now. Liang-ch'i had gone to study abroad. And his little sister was married. Ching-min lied and said she was married in order to save face.

Liang-san stared at her and asked, "Was that your son?"

"Yes," replied Ching-min, half in jest.

Liang-san looked pained, and, after a struggle, said regretfully, "Who'd have thought you could give birth to a son!"

The three other women at the table, Liang-san's wife and daughters, sat there quietly in a daze. Ching-min understood what it was like to be Liang-san's wife. She felt sorry for that woman. Wearing a plain, neutral-colored dress, she sat there quietly and obediently. When she met Liang-san she had been the most popular dancing girl in the music hall. One could still tell she was beautiful, but she looked a bit faded. It was as if that woman had taken Ching-min's place by Liang-san's side and gone on living in a quiet, faded, content manner. Maybe she was also happy that way. Ching-min hadn't had such a bad life before. But because of that woman she now was living a different kind of life. She felt she was better off now than before. She smiled at his wife good-naturedly but couldn't help joking, "Does he still hate to brush his teeth before going to bed?"

Liang-san and his wife blanched. He laughed, but she became angry. Maybe she wasn't as gentle as she seemed on the surface. This time she was herself, not like the former Ching-min. And she didn't feel like she was going to cry. Maybe she'd pick a fight with Liang-san when they went back home.

Ching-min went back to Liu Fen at the counter and had the kitchen make a special dish for Liang-san and his wife. As she headed for the kitchen, a cloud of steam came floating toward her. The chef in his white apron, the shiny stainless steel cabinets—perhaps this was the same impression from many years ago. Why were restaurant kitchens always the same? But she was not the same. She was now an independent, confident woman.

    * Yuan Chiung-Chiung 袁瓊瓊, *Ziji de tiankong* 《自己的天空》 (*A Place of One's Own*) (Taipei: Hongfan Press, 1981).

NOTES

1. *San* 三 is three in Chinese. The brothers in this story have been given names according to their seniority. Liang-ssu 四 is fourth brother; Liang-ch'i 七 is seventh brother.

CHAPTER 9

SEED OF THE RAPE PLANT

油蔴菜籽

Liao Hui-ying 廖輝英

(Translated by Chen I-djen 陳懿貞)

When Keke, my older brother, was born, my father was only twenty-three, and my mother was not quite twenty-one. She had attended a school for brides in Japan, and her dowry was twelve gold bars, twelve big trunks full of silk and woolen material, and many pieces of top quality furniture, brought over in a black sedan and trucks.

Black Pussy Cat, the doctor's youngest daughter, was finally getting married. In those days perfection such as hers was eyed with envy; her beauty and her family background brought out droves of matchmakers from nearby towns and villages, and many a young doctor had been turned down. Now she was finally getting married. What caused eyebrows to lift was that the groom was neither a doctor by profession, nor did he have the same social or economic background. He was only the son of a schoolteacher from a neighboring town and a graduate from a technical college. According to reports, the doctor liked him because he looked like a simple and honest man, and the young man's head of prematurely white hair, casually groomed, made him look much more honest and reliable than those fashionable doctors wearing French hairdos and Western-style clothing.

A year after the wedding they had a boy, which pleased the maternal grandfather so much that he could hardly keep his mouth closed from too much grinning. He had taken six concubines in succession, and still had not been able to produce a son. This event was a disappointment and a great let down to many who had been hoping that Black Pussy Cat's marriage would come up short.

I do not know how long the happy days lasted. I only know that as long as I could remember, Keke and I often had to hide in the corner watching our father throwing things around furiously, left and right. Mama would be screaming loudly, calling upon heaven and earth, her hair in great disarray. Quite a few times Mama left home after a big battle, while Keke and I, who had long ago learned to be alert to expressions on the faces of adults and to not cry easily, were hastily packed off to stay with Aunt Fu. Three or four days later our old, white-haired grandfather would bring our resentful mother back. Our father, who was never a man of words, was speechless before Grandfather, who was himself not a man of many words. The two of them would sit by the door in the setting sun, wordless. The old man, who had great wealth and great influence and whose face was heavily lined, no longer looked awe-inspiring, but was a picture of senility in the setting sun. To the son-in-law, the old man's quietude was not so much a reprimand as a request that he be good to his youngest and spoiled daughter. However, the tight-mouthed young man was no longer the simpleton who had panicked and sat on a washbasin when he was being looked over before the marriage.

I held on to my mother's skirt as we dragged ourselves to the black sedan parked at the entrance to the village to see Grandfather off. Our aged grandfather turned around and, looking at his daughter, said with a sigh, "Kitty, the fate of a woman is like a seed of the rape plant. A father can only try to make a selection that, hopefully, would be right for you, but, unexpectedly, after all that picking, we got one like him. Your papa's love for you turned out to be your undoing. It is your destiny. Your old father is over seventy, and will look after you in his remaining years. Your husband is not like your father. There's no way that he would spoil you lovingly as your father did."

When we got back home Papa had already left. Mama held me in her arms and said to Keke, sobbing broken-heartedly, "My silly boy, do you think that your mama really has no place to go? Your mama has one foot inside the door and one foot outside. She cannot take a step because of you children."

Situations like this, with mother and children crying in each other's arms, often happened in our younger days. In those days maybe we only wailed from panic and fear, when we saw her crying. How could we understand how a woman felt, sobbing away in a corridor, holding two young children in her arms during the twilight hours of the day?

The year after Titi, my kid brother, was born, our grandfather, who had been sickly for a long time, passed away. Mama practically crawled back to her father's house all the way from the bus station, wailing as she did so. On the day of the funeral our father took the three of us and milled around among the relatives in a state of stupor as our mother cried her heart out. I was used to her crying, but that time she did not cry in the same way as she did after a fight with our father. It was a soulful cry, as if she had lost her only support in this whole wide world, and even Grandfather's widows had to come over and comfort her.

Our father wore the mourning of a son-in-law, but he seemed absent-minded in contrast to our mother, who was sprawled out on the floor. He also had no patience with us. When our kid brother, Titi, would not stop crying, he cursed him with a few choice four-letter words. That day I followed him around timidly the whole day. Sometimes he walked too fast, and I did not dare to tug at his pants to slow him down. Later it often came to me that in those days Papa did not belong to us. He was all for himself. He tried to live the good life of a bachelor, which he missed. Nevertheless, he was the father of three. Maybe many times he forgot that he was.

But didn't he sometimes think of us? In those days when he was rushing about and was seldom home, he, to my surprise, brought me a big doll with fluttering eyes. When he waved that golden-haired doll and bade me to come to him, I could only stand at a distance, watching that big man who was a stranger. I was full of fears and doubts. The expression on his face then must have been sympathetic, otherwise how could I remember, after so many years, how he patiently coaxed his startled young daughter to accept his generous gift in that old thatch-roofed house in the country?

When I was six I attended the free kindergarten run by the factory for family of staff and workers, and I had to take Titi along. He attended the lower class, and I the upper class. At home I helped my mother to do chores such as washing the rice before cooking, wiping all the tatami floor mats, or playing with hateful Titi. On rare occasions my mother would look at me and say, "Ah-hui is a good girl. Children from hard-up families are more mature. Who else can help your ill-fated mother but you? Your older brother is a boy. He plays all day long and is not the least bit aware of the suffering of his mother."

Actually I was very envious of Keke. I thought he had a happier childhood. At least he was able to stay out of the house and play all kinds of games with his friends day in and day out. He had no patience with Titi, the crybaby. He hit him when he cried, therefore Mama never asked him to look after Titi. And what's more, he was luckily never home when Papa and Mama fought. He would either be out frolicking or sound asleep and could not be disturbed by anything. I was always the timid one. I could not let go, I could not leave Mama and Titi behind, I could not be like other village kids frolicking around in the orchard or in the planting field as if I had no worries and no cares.

Keke seemed to have no fear of Papa. Honestly, I think he came from the same kingdom as Papa. When Papa came home he usually brought him such magazines as *Oriental Youth* or *School Chums*. He was the king among the village kids, and they all played up to him because he lent those magazines out. One time Mama hit him. He cried and said, "So you hit me. I'm going to tell Papa to beat you up."

Mama hit him harder and cursed him between breaths, "You are a short-lived, unfilial son. I carried you for ten months and gave birth to you, and you have the nerve to say that you would ask your shameless father to beat me up. I'll kill you first." As she hit him again and again she started to wail.

When I was seven I went barefoot to the only elementary school in the village. I was not the only barefoot child in my class, so I was not especially concerned. But in the second term I was elected class president, and I was embarrassed to stand barefoot at the front of our class line-up. Moreover, all the other barefoot children were from farming families. I went home and told Mama, "The teacher said Papa is a mechanical engineer. We are not poor, and I ought to be given a pair of shoes. She also said that it's dangerous to cross the irrigation ditches unshod. There are watersnakes and wild plants that could hurt a person."

Mama said nothing. That night, after supper, after she put my one-year-old sister, Meimei, to sleep, she told me to put my feet on a piece of cardboard and traced the size and shape of my feet with a pencil. She then picked up a package wrapped in purple cloth and told me, "Ah-hui, Mama is going to Taichung. You go to bed. When Mama comes back she will have a pair of cotton shoes for you."

I pointed at the wrap and asked her, "What's that?"

"Something Ah-kung, your grandfather, gave Mama. Mama is going to sell it and buy you shoes."

That evening I tried to stay up in anticipation, half of me wanting to believe in her, half in doubt. I struggled hard to keep my eyes open while listening for passing buses on the only highway. Finally I dozed off into a fitful sleep.

When I woke up the next morning there was a pair of maroon shoes beside my pillow. I put them on proudly and walked back and forth on the tatami mats. What was more exciting was that breakfast was not the usual gruel but a piece of red bean paste bread from the store Yi Fu Tang. I ate it slowly, peeling off small pieces of the outside layers until there was only the small center ball of red bean paste left. Then I ate it lingeringly.

Ever since that time, Mama regularly took things out of her trunk and went to Taichung in the evening. The next day each of us would always have a piece of red bean paste bread. Moreover, tasty dishes would appear on the dinner table for a few days thereafter. Mama never failed to take an opportunity such as these to lecture me. "Ah-hui, you're a girl. You'll have to manage a household in the future. Mama will give you a few pointers. Go to the marketplace at noontime when the peddlers are about to call it a day. That's when you can get things cheap. If fate smiles on you, so be it, otherwise you'll have to know how to manage."

Gradually, Papa came home more often; still, he regularly went to Taichung after work. He'd come home and tidy up, and leave. He still screamed at Mama at the top of his voice, loudly and rudely, in our two-room apartment. They had no patience for one another. In those years it was a luxury for them to converse quietly and softly. They had been raising the roof for such a long time, it was hard to tell whether they were quarreling or not. But a picture of our Papa's furious face, the sound of our Mama's shrill voice, and a picture of him throwing her on the floor, punching and kicking her, appeared in front of our eyes again and again.

Thus, the days crept by slowly. One day Mama took one look at Papa's pay envelope and threw it on the tatami floor right then and there, and cursed in a loud voice, "You shameless four-legged beast! What else are you good for besides keeping that cheap woman? If your four kids had to depend on you, they would have long been starved to death. Out of a salary of over one thousand dollars only two hundred dollars is left!

How can I feed the four of them with that? When you're with your cheap woman, did you ever think of your children who are about to die of starvation? What disgrace! Supporting another's wife! Are those SOBs yours? Don't tell me that these four are not yours."

They cursed at one another. My younger brother and sister and I would make ourselves small in a corner. Suddenly Papa got hold of a meat cleaver and threw it at Mama. The cutting edge landed on Mama's ankle. For a split second, all was still until bright red blood started to gush out, looking like countless poisonous snakes crawling on Mama's white foot. I cried out in fear. My brother and sister started to holler too. Papa took a look at the three of us and left the room in anger, slamming the door behind him. Mama did not cry. She looked for cigarette butts, opened them up, threw away the wrapper, and applied the tobacco to the wound to stop it from bleeding.

That night I felt very cold. I kept dreaming of Mama all covered with blood. I cried and screamed, and promised to avenge her.

When I was promoted to the second grade, I still stood at the top of my class, and I was also designated the model student. My classmate Ah-chuan, who also lived in our village, told fellow classmates, "Li Jen-hui's father is a bad man. He's the lover of a woman in our village. How can she be a model student?"

I took off the round button given to model students and hid it in my school bag. I did not wear it again that term, and I never spoke to Ah-chuan again after that. I still wore my maroon-colored cloth shoes, now gaping open at the toes, and I still went through the planting field on my way to school, swinging a rice stalk in my hand. But how I wished I could leave this place, this place where there was a bad woman and a schoolmate who bad-mouthed me behind my back. Surely, there must be a place where no one knew about Papa. I would take Mama there with me.

One night I was awakened from my sleep by strange sounds. I opened my eyes and heard the terrible noise of a raging storm blowing against the roof tiles, and, from beyond the bamboo fence, the rain hitting against the branches and trees. Beside me, Keke, Titi, and Meimei were sleeping soundly. I heard Mama calling me in the dark in a soft voice. I crawled over Keke, Titi, and Meimei, and knelt beside her. With great effort she said, "Ah-hui, the baby in Mama's tummy is dead. I'm bleeding nonstop. Go get Aunt Chen and Aunt Fu to come and help. Do you dare to go? I wanted to wake up your older brother, but he's fast asleep, and I can't wake him."

Mama's face was icy cold. She told me to get her another deck of toilet paper. I rolled off the bed. Suddenly I feared that Mama was going to die. I said to her in a loud voice, "Mama, you mustn't die. I'll go get them, but you must wait for me."

I threw a raincoat over myself and went out barefoot. The eucalyptus trees swaying back and forth all over the village sounded like witches laughing. When I came to the ground for sunning grain, I ignored Ah-chuan's stories of ghosts and dashed across it. I fell and thought the ghosts were after me. I picked myself up and ran on. The raindrops hit my eyes and hurt so much that I could not keep them open. I stumbled all the way to the Fus' house and knocked on the door with all my might. Aunt Fu told me to go to the Chens' and ask Aunt Chen to go back with me and help while she went for the doctor.

I then ran through another half of the village to the Chens' residence. As I ran headlong into the bamboo fence, their big dog barked at me furiously from its cage. Aunt Chen waited until I finished my message, picked up a flashlight, put on her raincoat, and followed me out.

"Poor, poor soul! Your dad is not at home?"

I shook my head, and she looked at me and shook hers too. Walking beside her I felt drained all of a sudden. I almost could not get back home.

After the doctor left, Mama finally fell into a deep sleep. Aunt Chen said to me, "Poor, ill-fated soul! What ill fortune to be married to such a husband! If it hadn't been for this eight-year-old girl, it would have been the end of her today." Then she added, "I wonder what that unconscionable husband is lusting after now."

I knelt beside Mama and touched her face with my hand to make sure that she was only sleeping. Aunt Fu took my hand away and said, "Ah-hui, your mother is all right. Go to sleep. I'll watch over her. You can relax."

Mama's face was ashen. I refused to go to the inside room to sleep but stubbornly sprawled out beside her and gazed at her. Somehow, however, I fell asleep.

That year on New Year's Eve, the traditional steamed cake was already made. Mama, while grumbling regretfully that the cake had not risen as much as it should, thus indicating that there was no hope of prosperity in the coming year, muttered softly to herself as she sharpened a knife to kill the cock we had saved for more than a year for this occasion. Just then four or five big fellows came by. Papa paled as he was summoned. They did not come into the house but sat by the door. They neither touched the tea Mama offered nor paid any attention to Mama's polite conversation. They just kept pressing Papa with questions:

"You're an educated person. How can you do such an awful thing?"

"How can you sleep with someone else's wife? What about the moral principles of this world?"

"Such behavior should be punished by crippling you."

While those men cursed angrily, Papa stayed on one side, head lowered. Mama too sat on the other side, her eyes red, muttering all the while to herself.

This went on the whole morning. I stayed in the backyard watching the big cock. He stood on his two strong legs and shook his long neck as he pecked on a shorter chicken. Well, he probably would not be killed today, otherwise Mama would at least give me a fat chicken wing. Very regretfully I turned to look at a group of turkeys that would not be ready for slaughtering until next July fifteenth at the earliest. Alas, it was New Year's Eve, but we would not be eating either chicken nor rice noodles, and the chance of our getting new clothes or new shoes was even more remote. When would those rude and crude people be leaving?

My unruly younger brother, Titi, began to sob. I was too hungry to bother with him. Besides, I felt like crying myself. So I stayed put. He started to holler. Keke covered his mouth with his hand, and Titi hollered even louder. Keke slapped him, which only resulted in Titi simply letting himself go and crying with all his might. This scared Meimei, who was lying quietly until then, and she started crying too.

Mama came and slapped Keke real hard and said to me angrily, "Ah-hui, are you dead?"

I had no choice but to climb onto the tatami mats and pick up Meimei. I in turn cursed our unruly Titi, "Are you dead, Ah-hsin?"

What kind of New Year's celebration was this?

While we were making such a ruckus the men stood up, and the leader among them said, "Two thousand dollars normally would be a mere opener considering the magnitude of this shameful affair. We would not have let you off so easy today if it hadn't been for your four children and that today is New Year's Eve. This affair should be put to an end with a certain grace. Tonight at seven o'clock we'll be waiting for you in my house. Don't forget to set off a string of firecrackers. If you're not on time, I'm afraid it won't be pleasant for you."

Papa and Mama knelt by the door watching them leave. Mama turned in to the house and walked straight to the kitchen. She picked up the freshly steamed New Year's cake and started to slice it. Papa stayed by the door for a while, then he timidly followed her into the kitchen and said, "The money for tonight, I have to have it somehow."

Mama's words came out like rushing water as she screamed back, "Have to have it? It was your doing; you try to end it yourself. You slept with the woman; you try to find the money to cover up your shame. You and your shameless lust! Does it matter if the children are starving to death? Are you a man or mouse?"

There was no stopping Mama once she started. She cursed him and cried and cursed some more. She took a long time slicing the cake, but she was not putting the slices into a pan. The stove door was still covered by a rag. If she did not uncover it soon the fire would not be hot enough for cooking, but she was so mad that I dared not remind her of it.

Finally the cake was fried. Mama then went through her trunk and searched for a long time. Red-eyed, she wrapped up a large bundle with a piece of cloth. Papa brought out his newly bought twenty-inch Phillips bicycle and was waiting for Mama at the door. Mama told Keke and me, "Ah-chiang, Ah-hui, Mama is going to sell some stuff and pawn the bicycle to pay those people. You two older ones have to look after the younger ones. If you're hungry you can have some cake. When Mama comes back, Mama will cook for you. Be good. Do you hear?"

I gazed after them as they left. I wanted to but dared not ask if the cock would be killed. I could merely bring myself to ask Keke, "What does 'pawn' mean?"

"Stupid! It means to sell. To sell something in exchange for money. That's what it means. Can't you even understand that?"

That day Papa and Mama came back very late. The cock, of course, was spared. We had salted gruel that evening. We did not go through the usual worship ceremony, so, of course, there were no special things to eat. But in the end the cock would not be able to escape its fate. It would be killed sooner or later. So thinking, I fell asleep with a ray of hope in spite of my disappointment at not getting any New Year's Eve money.

After school started, Mama went there to get a transfer for Keke and me. We were going to leave this place. I was so happy that I forgot my vow and ran up to Ah-chuan and said to him bluntly, "We're moving to Taipei."

The startled and stupid look on his face pleased me to no end. I ran away thinking to myself that he was nothing but a smelly boy who liked to bad-mouth others.

We moved to Taipei and rented a house from my Aunt Tsui-hung. Mama kept the big chickens and the native chickens near the water pump, and she also bought some American broilers. It was said that this kind of fowl grew fast, and would start to lay eggs in four months. Soon we would be eating exorbitantly expensive eggs without having to spend any money at all.

Papa bought a second-hand bicycle and rode it back and forth to work. He got home early those days. An easel was set up in the living room. When he had time he often put on his shorts and started to paint, using many different colors. Our neighbors sometimes asked for his paintings. He got carried away and painted more and more. Although Mama did not tell him not to paint, she usually commented contemptuously, "What good is it? It'll not bring any money for food." Sometimes when she was in a foul mood she'd say, "Other husbands think of ways to make money to bring food to the table so that their wives and children can have good lives. Your old dad only brings back his monthly salary, which is not enough to make ends meet."

Be that as it might, I was happy to see Papa home regularly, and, furthermore, he fought less with Mama. He seldom talked to me. I thought he probably did not know how to talk to me. I had always, since infancy, watched him from a distance. But he would often take Titi by the hand and, carrying Meimei with his other arm, go buy the kind of steamed cake that cost ten cents each piece, and he never failed to bring back one piece each for Keke and me.

Keke and I both attended the elementary school across the bridge; he in the fifth grade, I in the third. In those days intensive tutoring started in the third grade. Some five or six members in the class had no intention of entering high school, and they had to help the teacher with odd jobs. The rest of our class all had to take part in a city-wide examination, therefore it necessarily followed that we had to take part in the intensive tutoring program, because many important subjects were taught only in the tutorial sessions.

After our transfer I realized that the teachers in Taipei based their assignments on reference books. In the country we had never even heard of the term "reference books." Reference books cost over ten dollars each. Keke was in a higher grade and closer to taking the city-wide examination, so he needed several each term. We could not afford to buy all the books needed, so Mama made the decision that his were given priority. Therefore for three or four weeks in a row, my teacher lashed the palm of my hand with a thick strip of rattan because I had not done my homework. Did the teacher think that this kid from the rural district was beyond help?

At the end of every month our teacher would announce, "Tutorial fees must be paid tomorrow." And the next day I would watch over sixty of my schoolmates lining up to pay. The going price then was thirty dollars a month. The rich students paid one or two hundred. I sat there shamefaced, watching the impressive line disperse, then I had to brace myself to sit through our teacher's proclaiming loudly the names of those who had not paid. For a week or two following this, names would be called every day until finally mine would be the only one called. I could not take it anymore, so I tried to discuss it with Mama. "I don't want to be tutored anymore."

"Isn't it true that many of the subjects are covered only in these tutorial sessions?"

I nodded and said, "I don't really have to take the examinations for junior high school."

"You want to have the kind of life your mama had?" Mama pulled a long face and lectured me sternly. "A woman with no skills will have to depend on her husband for a living. If she marries well, then it's her good fortune, so be it. If she marries an irresponsible fellow, what's she going to do for food? Eat sand? Your mama is not exactly unschooled. I even went to Japan for a few years of schooling. Didn't I have a good life when I was young? But I married and had children, and it finished me. I didn't go out to work, and the second half of my life just can't be compared with others."

"But," I said haltingly, fingering the corner of my skirt, "Not paying the tutorial fee, my name is called every day, and they all turn and look at me as if I were a freak."

"In a couple of days I'll try to manage for you to pay. Mama will manage to get twenty dollars."

"All the others pay thirty; that's the minimum."

"Be happy that we can pay this much. That it is ten dollars less cannot be helped. So we are poor!"

My monthly tutorial fee was met in this dragged-out manner. Often times I no sooner paid one month's expense when the other students would be beginning to pay for the following month's. The shame I had to suffer for having my name announced in our classroom and for the sidelong looks of my fellow students were compensated for by the honor of always being among the top of my class in every monthly examination.

The next year Keke was 1.5 points short and could only go to the school of his second choice. It was regrettable, but I think Mama was, nonetheless, pleased. He was her first-born. For a child from the country who had nothing to do with tutoring and reference books until the second term of his fifth grade year to squeeze through the narrow portals of a provincial junior high school was something that made even our ever-lukewarm papa, who never bothered with his children, happy. However, in order to meet the tuition for the provincial high, which was over two hundred dollars, and to manage the additional tens of dollars for uniforms, Mama was really squeezed. Papa buried his head like an ostrich as if all this had nothing to do with him. Mama could scream all she wanted as she walked in and out of the house, calling him "useless" at the top of her voice for the thousandth time; he would still stay in his corner and paint his pictures as if nothing had happened.

In those years Mama got up at the break of dawn to start a fire outdoors. She first used a few sheets of paper from our old exercise books, on top of which she then piled a few pieces of thinly sliced tinder and finally some briquettes. When we got up there would be two bowls of freshly cooked rice waiting for us. In the bowl for Keke there were two eggs. I got only one.

Mama's explanation for this discrepancy was that Keke was a boy—he was growing, he ate more rice, therefore he had an extra egg.

Once I ate that part of the rice mixed with egg and refused to eat the little bit of plain rice left in the bowl. Mama scolded me, "What a waste! Ah-hui? Do you know how much is a catty of rice?"

"Why can't I have two eggs?" I muttered. "It's I who clean the chicken droppings every night. Keke never has to clean up after them."

Mama was taken aback. After a long pause she said, "Why are you haggling? A woman's fate is like a seed of the rape plant: it grows where it falls. The good fortune of an unmarried woman does not count. Mama is fair. Poor as we are, I let you go to school. In another family you would have been sent away to work as a housemaid long ago. Your older brother will have to carry on the Li family line. Why are you bargaining tit for tat? Who knows what name you're going to take later on?"

Mama lowered her voice gradually, picked up the dishes, and went back in.

After that I learned to eat my bowl of rice and one egg wordlessly, and I no longer complained that I had to do so many chores after my tutorial session, while Keke could swim all he wanted or play basketball, and that he didn't even have to do the dishes.

I had a lot of homework in the two years before the city-wide examination. In school I dutifully did my work, but after school I only did my homework; I no longer dug into my books. Whenever I recalled how the household was turned topsy-turvy over even the registration fee and how Mama had to struggle to meet monthly household expenses and Keke's tuition, I decided deep down in the bottom of my heart that if I did not pass, I would just quit school.

In the sixth grade I entered a school-wide art competition and won first prize, a box of twenty-four watercolors and two brushes. I showed them at home, extremely pleased with myself. Mama, who was in the middle of doing the dishes, rolled her eyes and said very sternly, "Do you think they're great? You'd be like your good-for-nothing Papa, paint and paint and paint. Did all that painting produce any wealth? You'd better give up this bad business right away."

I never thought that Mama could get so mad and that I would be the object of her scorn. The prize, something I could never afford, turned sour. After that I never talked about it when I entered composition competitions or poster competitions. In those days, when I came home with my report cards, Mama would look at them and put her seal on them. She never asked how come I was the second in my class that month, nor did she utter any encouragement when I was the top of my class. I thought, *So what if I did well or poorly! No one cared.* That being the case I no longer took the extra tutorial sessions in the evening, yet I still remained within the top three of my class.

The day the results of the city-wide examination for junior high were out, Mama woke me up from my afternoon nap and snapped, "Did you die in your sleep? The radio has been announcing the results the whole afternoon. Bet you did not pass. If so, see if you can still sleep as soundly as a pig."

I rolled out of bed and stood by the door of a neighbor's to listen to the broadcast. I stood there so long that I thought my legs were going to break. They were still announcing the names of the boys. I neither dared go back home nor did I have any idea how long I had to wait. While I was hesitating I saw Papa came back on his bicycle. He yelled happily before he reached our door, "You passed! You passed!"

Mama came out from the house and said anxiously but angrily, "Of course she passed. The question is which school."

"Her first choice. I was sure it would be her first choice." Papa parked his bicycle and gestured for me to go to him, looking extremely pleased. "The list was published in the paper. Do you have any idea how long it would be before you'd hear it on the radio?"

Those were probably my best and my most glorious days. Papa, who never dwelt on things concerning me, was inexplicably happy. He told people repeatedly, "She scored quite a few points above the admission score. Got twenty-five points for composition, a real high score."

Was Mama also pleased? She never told anybody and kept busy as always. I was not spared any of my chores as a result of the examinations.

It was at this time that Papa got some side jobs doing mechanical drawings. He did not negotiate about payment. Mama blamed him for not knowing how to haggle, and he would reply, very sure of himself, "It won't happen; it won't happen! People will not shortchange us."

As it turned out, after burning the midnight oil for a few nights, he was completely taken aback by the meager sum they paid him. After that he was no longer enthusiastic about that kind of job.

Papa took a day off on registration day and took me to school on his bicycle. We had to spend the entire morning lining up in the auditorium, going to one desk after another. I did not know what happened to Papa, but he seemed to be unable to stop himself from talking to other parents in the line. The conversation was about how many points the other children got, or which elementary school they were from. Whenever he found someone with grades lower than mine, he would be pleased beyond words and say, "See! Quite a few points lower; almost had to take second choice." When I was being measured for my uniform, he was even more excited and said repeatedly, "In all of Taipei only your school issues this kind of uniform."

That day for lunch, Papa treated me to a bowl of beef noodles and gave me five dollars and told me, "Don't tell your old mom about it. We'll charge this against registration fees."

I did feel guilty cheating my extremely thrifty mama, but, when I thought of my papa, who had always been hard up and who now at long last had an opportunity to show his daughter a childlike sincere concern, I had to keep quiet. After school started Papa was more interested in my schoolwork than I was. Whenever I picked up my English textbook, he would say, in a very high spirit, "Come! Papa will help you." He would pick up the textbook and read on and on, unmindful of anything else, in a Japanese accent, until Mama gave it to him: "Crazy! The girl is studying, and you are disturbing her. She has an exam tomorrow morning. Do you know about that?"

Papa was most interested in helping me with my homework during those junior high school years. His favorite statements in those days were, "Ah-hui is like me," or "Ah-hui has beautiful penmanship, like me." The gist of it was that anything good about me I took from him. Mama would always mercilessly pour cold water on him: "Heaven forbid! Worst fate if she is like you."

Papa probably was quite happy with himself in those years. He often gave me a few dimes when no one was looking and indicated that I should not mention it to anybody. I saw him hide a few dollars clumsily in his shoe, and I predicted that they would be discovered by Mama. And they were. From then on he began hiding money all over in places he thought were very safe. Maybe he was in too much of a hurry when he hid it, or maybe he moved it around so often that he would forget where it was, so that later when he looked for his stashes he could not find them. He would end up sweating profusely and, braving the danger of Mama's scorn, would have to ask her. The end result was either we all had to help him look, or it would cause another rowdy quarrel. At any rate his private savings would automatically go to the treasury. Therefore I was well aware that he always kept some money for himself to buy a pack of cigarettes or to hand out a few dimes secretly to us kids, but I never could bring myself to tell Mama. Was it because he was so childlike? Was it because I realized that one should not have designs on such a naive person? I kept quiet.

He might have been able to manage a continuous flow of petty cash, but registration time was always an embarrassing moment for Papa. When pressed, Mama told us to ask Papa for money. His usual answer was, "Ask your old mama."

"Mama told us to ask you."

"Where would I get the money? I gave her all my salary. I don't know how to produce gold."

Should we press further, he would lose his temper and say, "Quit school then, since there's no money."

It was frustrating and it repeated itself time and again. However, it made us feel that Papa was a caged beast who could not find a way out. He was a free soul and fit only to lead a carefree life by himself. To burden him with the responsibility of being the head of a household only made him look inadequate. He married too young. It was the same with our mama, whose dreams were shattered too early in her life. The two of them each cherished their own wild dreams, and neither knew how to deal with the crude realities of married life.

The years went by, at times submitting to fate; at times rebelling noisily against it. Mama was pregnant again with my youngest brother, Hsiao-ti, at thirty-seven. Every day her protruding silhouette would waddle all around the house with a heavy heart, either squatting under the faucet doing the laundry or taking care of this or that. Just before the baby was born, I brought out my piggy bank, which contained my two years of savings, from where it was hidden under my bed. I handed it to Mama silently. She handed me a rusty axe and said, "The money is yours. You break it yourself."

Even before she had finished speaking, she started crying.

With one stroke I broke the bank, and dimes flew all over the floor. My young dream of joining a hiking trip across the East-West Cross-Island Highway was also shattered. Then, mother and daughter sat across from one another in a dark corner in the kitchen silently piling up the dimes: one, two...

Why was life like that?

After graduation from junior high, I passed the entrance examinations to both the senior high school and the normal school for girls. Mama insisted that I go to the normal school. She said, "It's free. Besides, what's the point of a girl having so much schooling? It's not as if you were planning to remain an old maid. A reliable job ought to be good enough for you."

I don't know whether it was because that was the first time I ever went against my mother and held firm to my idea, or because, starting with that year, Papa was engaged to work in the Philippines and earned a salary much greater than before, but, in any event, Mama eventually agreed to allow me to continue on to senior high.

Those years were quite the opposite of the bad years in the past. The days seemed to go by smoothly and quickly. Papa was far away in a foreign land, and he kept a part of his salary to enable him to once again live the good life of a bachelor. Distance also seemed to have eased the sharp conflicts between them, now separated by mountains and seas. Every week he sent back loving words showing his concern and longing. He even carefully referred to every member of the family. Occasionally he sent us gifts through people returning from that distant land, specifying which was for which. They were for the most part not very practical items. He also carefully wrapped up clothing he bought for us in sizes he imagined us to be and sent them by air. All this was done by the same pair of hands that had beaten us as well as guided us.

Mama sometimes grumbled about his unforgivable past; at other times she looked forward to his letters and gifts, always half-complaining and half-smiling in a helpless manner. But who wanted to find fault with this kind of life? We now even had money for non-essentials, and she no longer had to wrack her brains for the small things in life.

But when I passed the entrance exams and was admitted to college, for which Mama had prayed and burned a stick of incense twice a day, once in the morning and once in the evening, she looked at the report card and said, the corners of her mouth drooping in a contemptuous manner, "The pig does not grow fat, but the fat grows on a dog."

This was truly a deflating statement to a girl's ego.

Then, she seemed to have forgotten her own words as she dashed about getting fresh flowers and fruit to spread on the sacrificial table. She told me to kneel down and kowtow twelve times. The clear outline of Mama's face looking solemn and kind, through the misty smoke of incense, watching me from above, looked very much like that of the Goddess of Mercy.

I remained my innocent self. I drifted along effortlessly. I neither fought for nor shied away from anything. Like the others, I also tutored children at their homes. I started to write articles to earn my own keep. In the four more or less uneventful college years, I kind of took on the responsibility of an older sister and mother. I looked after a string of younger brothers and sister, while Mama started to go to the temple religiously. She became a vegetarian and semi-retired housewife. All worldly affairs concerning sons and daughters automatically became my inherent duty.

Papa's glorious years were over. When he returned home he had long passed employment age. He was able to find stable jobs only because of his technical knowledge and experience, but he probably found them unfulfilling. He appeared to be inconsistent and changeable. Sometimes, on his way back from work when he had to change buses he would go to the Buddhist temple to buy an order of diet noodles for Mama. He would show great concern and urge her to eat it while it was still hot. At other times he might have a fit of temper because she had gone to the temple to have a dietary meal. At such times he would act as if he was going to break each and every one of the idols on the sacrificial table. Sometimes he could be very patient and explain to Mama, sentence by sentence, the foreign or Mandarin-language movies on television. At other times he would ridicule her for not even knowing how to take a bus or to manage basic Mandarin. Mama still talked the way one chopped wood, splitting the wood with one sweep of the axe mercilessly and uncompromisingly. Time and again she told, in great details, of our father's misdeeds. Papa, on the other hand, showed that he was most unhappy with the fact that Mama could not find a job and share his burden. One of them was now an old man whose back was bent, whose hair was graying, and whose teeth were loose. The other was a housewife who had spent thirty years making ends meet, an old woman whose hair had turned gray and whose sight was failing. Yet the frequency and the intensity of their fights were as bad as they were in their younger days. After thirty years of a hard life, and after all the years of going at one another, they still had not learned to coexist without animosity. Hadn't they paid a price for all this? And all those hurts, were they injuries that could not be compensated for?

In those days Keke was unwilling to follow Papa's footsteps in a salaried job. He tried to set up a business from scratch. It bled him dry, and he had no time for the family. That responsibility automatically became mine. For a few years after my graduation, I was able to get a fairly high salary, earned through blood and sweat. Maybe I was lucky; maybe I was driven by a stubborn desire to make something of this family. At any rate, I worked hard and moonlighted, holding a few side jobs. I made quite a bit of money through the years. Our home suddenly looked a lot different.

After making my way for a few years, I, who had always been placid, now displayed an excitable characteristic. In the business corporation where the hens contended to rule the day, I was sometimes unable to fend for myself. The kind of life I lived before, drifting effortlessly as fate dictated, now seemed far, far away.

Mama had changed too. Maybe she was only reverting to her old self before her marriage, maybe she was trying to recoup from her thirty anemic years, but she had suddenly become very demanding now, very hard to please. The difference in her between now and then could even be seen in the way she dressed. In the old days, so that her children could have what they needed, she went unkempt, her face unwashed, and she never had a new dress from one year to another. She had even been mistaken for a kitchen maid. Now, whenever I went shopping with her she picked only Swiss or Japanese imported material. The fabrics I picked to have dresses made to wear to work every day were too ordinary for her. Thus, after a few such shopping sprees, I was considered a favorite customer. When the stores received new merchandise they never failed to call me at my office. I did what I could, figuring I had boundless amounts of energy and that money may go out one way, but it will come back again. And indeed, I felt that Mama really had gone through a lot in the past. Would it be possible to give her another thirty years? Whatever I could do, why should I be stingy about it? Thus, season after season, I would always take along large rolls of money and pay for her selections generously.

Mama could not go shopping by herself, so I shopped not only for her but also for things like shirts, pants, sweaters, and vests for Papa. I had to guess at the size and buy accordingly. Mama considered herself somewhat above all worldly cares. She had long ago relinquished her control over many practical but miscellaneous matters, though she was never able to shake off such worldly sentiments as love and hate, or anger and scorn. Therefore, each time I bought a dress for myself I never forgot to buy one for Meimei too. I was a typical housewife in those days. I not only had to look after everyday matters such as clothing, food, living, and transportation expenses, but also to coerce my younger brothers and sister to take all sorts of lessons after school. I was so afraid that they would grow up like me, good at nothing else but schoolwork, and that they would become too uptight and dull. I even worried that they might not be able to master any one skill, and also urged them to learn more in other fields of work. Was it because in my day I was never able to get anything I wanted and that I missed too much, so that now when I could afford it, I urged them on my sister and brothers like an old mother? Come to think of it, deep down in me, did I also have the same fear as Mama?

Under the circumstances, how could one not try to make as much money as one could?

As for Mama, I did not know whether poverty had instilled a permanent fear in her or she had reached a mental state of greediness. She was constantly complaining to me of being poor. She sometimes praised the children of our acquaintances and spiced it up by saying how able and filial they were. Reading between the lines, I seemed to be most lacking in every way.

A few years back I underwent major surgery and was bedridden for forty days. My surgical expenses were paid by friends. Only then, when neither my body nor my soul was at my command, did I realize what a dreadful state it was not having any savings. At that point I began to join a hui[1] in the company behind Mama's back. She, however, cleverly suspected it and tried to find out more as best she could. She was most unhappy about my secret savings. At that time her own private savings amounted to hundreds of thousands, but she did not keep it in a savings bank. She locked it up in her cabinet. She worshipped money. Should anyone in the family, with the exception of Keke, ask her for money, he or she would necessarily get a good scolding. In the end, she would give, but less than asked for. She was also likely to throw the money into the far corner of the room for the asker to pick up.

In those years her temper worsened as our family condition improved. One or another of us, young or old, could be the cause of her displeasure.

She would curse us in a shrill voice, going from room to room. She was sometimes really unreasonable.

The young ones were likely to argue with her after an exchange of no more than two or three words. Once she got started, Mama would cry and complain about her fate, tears rolling down her face, her nose running. If any one of us went against her, she would go all the way back and enumerate all the things that each member of the family had done. Not one of us was spared, and this would go on for days. I really dreaded the way she went on day and night, night and day, so I would scold whoever went against her. I had also learned to let it all go in one ear and out the other, and I never talked back. My brothers and sister blamed me for spoiling her, and they made fun of me, saying that I was "stupidly filial." They said it made them look unfilial by comparison. However, considering all that had happened in the past, why could we not let her have her way now? We all owed her that much.

In those ten years she disapproved of all the people I associated with. She was sometimes rude to them over the phone, and sometimes kept visitors waiting outside in the rain. On the rare occasions when I came home late she would not let anyone open the door for me. She made me stand in the pitch-dark alley listening to her obscene cursing drifting down from the fourth floor apartment. I was already an adult over twenty. Surely she loved me in spite of her ways! When any of the others went against her she would suddenly remember that only this daughter knew about her pain. Even though I seldom ate at home, when she went shopping for food she invariably remembered to buy some kidneys for me. Many nights when I was exhausted and ready to drop off she would walk into my room to chat about this and that. At such times I seemed to see the face of a loving mother, bearing a resemblance to the Goddess of Mercy, the one who looked down upon me as I lit the incense and kowtowed after I passed the college entrance examinations.

Actually, I wasn't really following her wishes in the matter of matrimony during those years. There was simply no one to rouse my interest.

I was merely exhausted. I only wanted to hide in a world where there were no quarrels and no hatred, and where I did not have to break my neck to get ahead. Mama again and again cited examples of marriage failures among friends and relatives as warnings. She was most emphatic about the incompatibility between Papa and her, who got along like fire and water. She said, "Not to get married is not necessarily a misfortune. A girl's fate is like that of a seed of the rape plant. If her marriage does not work she will be stuck with it the rest of her life. This is the way with your mama. Look at you now, you dress nicely and go to work every day, and there's no need for you to wait on anybody. Now, what's wrong with that? Why should you want to get married?"

After thirty years of tears, Mama was constantly in a deep abyss of fear. In her twilight years she became a devout Buddhist and courted fate, but still things were not going as well as she would have liked. Everything irritated her: my brothers' careers, the friends they kept, and their marriages, but more than anything else, none of her three sons stayed with her, the sons whom she expected to continue the family line. They left home because they could not put up with the atmosphere at home. As far as she was concerned, a daughter was only a daughter no matter how good she was. Only the sons could keep the Li family incense burning. She had no praise and no respect for marriage.

Unfortunately it was at this time that I made my decision about marriage. To my surprise, she did not object strenuously. Maybe she was tired, maybe it was because of my insistence. But when she finally nodded feebly as if she had no alternative, I suffered a feeling of regret. When the final decision was made she iterated time and again, "For better or for worse, it's your fate. You made the choice yourself."

The wedding ceremony was hastily arranged. I did not really care about the ritualistic formalities. However, when Mama showed the fortuneteller our pa-tzu, the eight characters denoting our time of birth—the year, the month, the day, and hour—she was told that the wedding date clashed with her horoscope. She could not personally see me off. She was deeply regretful about that.

"The Goddess of Brides rules supreme. I must stay away. I brought this girl up yet I cannot see her in her wedding gown. I raised a good daughter and can't even see her out of our door. It's really not worthwhile."

The fact that Mama could not send me off in my white veil saddened me even more than her. She had sheltered me under her wing through many difficult decades and made me what I was. She should be seeing me off personally no matter what. In my opinion, supreme as the Goddess of the Brides might be, she could not possibly overshadow a mother.

Mama, however, preferred to believe in it.

On the eve of my wedding day I put on my wedding dress for Mama alone. She stooped down on the floor of the apartment where we had lived for over ten years, feeling the white veil on the floor with her hand while looking up at this seed of rape plant that was about to fall into an unknown field.

I touched her graying hair with my gloved hand. She looked so helpless in the mirror, so old and feeble as if she were unable to negotiate the distance to see where this rape seed was going to land. I fell down on my knees. For the first time in my life I held her in my arms, with her face pressed against my white-veiled breast. I wanted very much to tell her that I would be happy, that she should put her heart at ease. But when I looked at that face that reflected the untold sorrow of the years past and saw how it had aged, I could only cry, "Mama, Mama!"

* This story was first published in the "In This World" 人間 section (ed. Kao Shang-chin 高上秦) of the *China Times* 中國時報 on October 6, 7, and 8, 1982, and it won the first prize in the short story contest.

NOTES

1. A *hui* is a group that collects money from its members at regular intervals, and members will in turn collect the pot.

Chapter 10

The Devil in a Chastity Belt

戴貞操帶的魔鬼

Li Ang 李昂

(Translated by Laura Jane Way 魏正儀)

I

In the very beginning it was just a picture, a picture in a travel magazine.

A portion of a statue could be seen in it: a coldly handsome man, his wavy hair slightly disheveled, his muscular body entirely bare except for a belt-like object with a triangular arrow curving from one side of his torso toward the front of his lower body, the arrow neatly obscuring his loins. The picture roused her interest, and, pointing to the arrow, she said to the man leafing through the magazine at her side, "What is this?"

"It's the devil," he replied, clearly amazed by her inability to identify him. "Don't you see that he has a pointed tail with a triangular arrow? See, he even has two horns on his head."

Only then did she see the protruding horns upon the head and the pointed tail with the arrow.

"This is what the devil looks like?" she said, her astonishment genuine.

They had come to attend a no-longer-secret meeting of blacklisted individuals in Europe. The ban on the blacklist had not yet been lifted the previous year when the meeting was being planned overseas, and dissenters were only able to return to their native land, after decades in exile, by surreptitious and often perilous means.

With the exception of a handful of these people, nobody knew for sure what the aforementioned "surreptitious means" were. However, it was commonly believed that as a result of the iron grasp of the dictatorship upon the island, the chances of lawfully entering the country though immigration were nil.

(There were people who had attempted to go through immigration, but they had all been deported. Not only were things tightly controlled on the island, but the overseas intelligence was also efficient. No wonder people whispered in private that everything would be prepared on the island to ensnare the dissenters in a ready-spun web the moment they stepped onto a plane.)

So the sea was the only possible means of return. Fly to the nearest Asian country, and from there, change to a small boat.

Despite its multitude of soldiers and secret police, the island country, surrounded on all sides by water, had a long, rugged coastline that no number of patrols could make impenetrable. A way home was thus left open to the exiles.

But the price of a blacklist homecoming could well be life itself.

Most often the only boats available were small smugglers' vessels, which could capsize at any moment. The greatest peril, however, lay in being arrested—in the confusion dissenters could conveniently be "mistaken" for smugglers and executed on the spot, after which excuses would be made about identification being impossible in the commotion, and so on and so forth. Therein lay the true danger of the journey.

Forever bound up with the name "smuggler," even in death.

But there were still people who managed to make their way home, despite the odds, although it was possible that countless days behind bars awaited them.

"Even if I should have to sit it out in jail, I'd be doing it in my own country, upon my own soil," declared those on the blacklist.

They were opposition-party congressmen from the island. She was a legislator, and he a people's representative. They had come to this old city in Europe for a no-longer-secret blacklist gathering.

The city, like so many old ones in Europe, had a river winding through it. Be it the blue Danube, the green Rhine, or some other river, the area through which the river flowed became the heart of the city, pulsating with life.

Where there were rivers, there were bound to be bridges linking the two banks. There wouldn't just be one bridge, but many: modern steel-and-concrete bridges for commuter trains, cars, and city-dwellers; steel bridges exclusively for trains; and of course an old, old bridge built hundreds of years ago, its heavy stone bulk spanning the serene-looking river. Steps were taken for its preservation—only pedestrians were allowed on the bridge, tourists making up the greater part of the throng.

The old bridge was known worldwide for the statues, mainly of several larger-than-life figures from the Bible and local lore, that lined its two sides. The two of them, like most tourists, gave the array of statues a cursory glance without taking particular pains to identify each and every one of them, feeling as though they were merely passing through a historical carnival parade. The pious deeds of saints, the blood-spattered glory of tyrants, the virtue of the pure were all but a backdrop for the romantic aspirations and aura of antiquity that travelers came in search of in the warmth of the European spring. The trees on the banks of the river were covered thickly with green leaves; flowers of all kinds dotted the emerald expanses of lawn on the levees; bushes of lilacs, long in bloom, infused the soft air with whiffs of mellow fragrance.

If only the effusive chairman of the European section wouldn't insist on accompanying them as they wandered through the crowds of souvenir vendors, magicians, and street musicians, chattering nonstop about possible political developments on the island!

The night they had arrived in the city, they checked into a hotel close to the old bridge. The bridge could be seen from the window of her room, brightly lit up by multi-colored lights like a boulevard of dreams arching over the water, lost in the darkness below. The lights of the castle, the town, and the palace on the opposite bank shone somewhat dimmer from a distance, creating an aura of mystery and enchantment, as though the city were one of elfin wonder, floating through the boundless scope of the night sky.

She invited him to her room to share this incredible view, for the room he was in did not face the bridge.

He accepted her invitation. Seating himself in her room, he resumed the discussion they had had with the chairman earlier that day about the migration of the organization to Taiwan. Then very soberly he said, "Seeing these overseas people and their affairs, and seeing Taiwan from afar on this trip has lent greater clarity to many things in my mind. There will be great changes in Taiwan in the years to come, and when people like us leave Taipei for even one short week, who we are and what we do may be of no consequence by the time we return."

He paused for a moment. Then, casting his usual caution aside, he said, "Look at these overseas people. Exiled decades ago, they've fought and struggled, made sacrifices, and given up so much. Now, finally, they are free to return home. But what is there for them to do back in Taiwan?"

He looked up at her, seeking feedback. He realized that she was not listening and, furthermore, couldn't care less.

"If this were Taipei with the same river and the same bridge, there would be no need to light the bridge up, for it would be futile. There would be people everywhere anyway, and lights: house lights and streetlights, or car lights and neon lights," she mused, sunk in thought, her expression indecipherable.

He looked at the blank mask upon her face, the face of the "Grieving National Mother" he had gotten so used to over the years. Suddenly he didn't know what to say.

Her husband was still in prison when she was elected legislator. She was a wife who carried on her husband's work in his stead, and the people supported her with their anonymous votes, giving her entrance to the legislature by a landslide. Before that, they had already elected her as people's representative in an effort to make it up to her outstanding, courageous husband, a member of parliament who had been sentenced to fifteen years in prison after the Big Arrest.

That very same husband had been known as "the Cannon" in the parliament.

As for her, she had been a pretty little wife, born on the island to a middle-class family and raised to be a high school music teacher. She had a son and a daughter, sweet as cherubs. Her skill with the violin —her major instrument—was neither better nor worse than that of the average student of music, but apart from that she also loved all that was beautiful: Japanese flower-arranging, tea-making, and literature.

Her home had been renowned for its daintiness. The country folk who used to come to see her husband hesitated to put the embroidered slippers she offered them onto their huge, toil-roughened feet, preferring to go barefoot. And they gulped down big mouthfuls of her Japanese green tea, which, according to them, "tasted like seaweed."

"There was a ring of foam on top, and it was said the finer the foam, the better," they said, bragging of the extraordinary hospitality they received in her home.

They all respected the gracious woman, often bowing deeply to her in apology for having to drag her husband into the dangers of opposition work, saying, "Makoto ni sumimasen (we are really sorry)." It was as though they had to apologize to her good upbringing, her violin, her flower-arranging, and her tea-brewing.

She was an ever-dutiful wife and mother, never interfering in her husband's political activities. Everyone knew that she had no interest whatsoever in politics, and would never have gotten caught up in the melee had she not fallen in love for the first time in college with the diligent law student from a farming village.

Would she ever stand in the way of her husband's opposition work for the sake of her young son and daughter and her lovely home, though?

Nobody openly discussed this. People spat betel-nut juice on the ground and said with gruff tenderness, "Well, she's a woman."

What they left unsaid was: "They're all like this."

The betel-nut juice issued from their mouths, spattered, bright red as blood, on the ground.

The husband had apparently never let the tender love of his little wife deter him. Perhaps it wasn't even necessary for him to do anything in the first place; the absolute power of the autocracy had to be secured through a continuous series of arrests of members of the opposition, and it was inevitable that the Cannon should be proclaimed a "traitor" and thrown into jail during that gory island-wide Big Arrest on Christmas Eve.

He would probably have been sentenced to death had it not been for the intervention of the international community and the aid from overseas. (Those who gave aid, if not already on the blacklist, would shortly be added to it because of this.) Having been exempted from the death penalty, some of those arrested were sentenced to life imprisonment, and the Cannon, although he had been absent from the site of the protest march that night, because he was entertaining members of a foreign observation group in secret, was sentenced to fifteen years in prison.

They had come all the way from the faraway island country to this lovely old city in Europe to attend a no-longer-secret blacklist meeting. The meeting had a beautiful name that was tinged with sadness: Home-coming of the Salmon.

It was he who had done everything in his power to work this trip to Europe into her tight schedule. Most of the overseas people who had provided her husband with unflagging support all these years, and who had gone to countless trouble to facilitate his release, were on the blacklist. She had to come in person, if only to express her gratitude toward them.

Moreover, the meeting was for planning the return of blacklisted individuals to their native land; these people, if they finally got to go home, could become invaluable to her camp.

Naturally, she agreed to come. From people's representative to legislator, she had been admired most for her sensitivity as a woman to the public relations of politics.

However, while the meeting was in the process of being planned, the dictator passed away. Though the reign of terror didn't disintegrate afterward as quickly as had been expected, it was beyond the power of the successor to resume the dictatorship, and so the grip on the blacklist loosened at last.

The hard work of the overseas dissenters finally paid off when, about a month before their planned trip to Europe, those on the second and third tiers of the blacklist became eligible to apply for visas from the home country. The visas usually didn't allow long stays—a week or two, one month at the very most—but they certainly revealed a promise of things easing up further in the future.

And so the secret meeting ceased to be a secret. The struggle these people were prepared to engage in, their determination to sacrifice their lives the way a salmon dedicates its life to returning to its birthplace—all this was no longer necessary. The committee accordingly altered the main objective of the meeting, concentrating now upon the journey back to Taiwan.

They had to decide whether or not to make the journey. She was determined to attend—"If just to show my gratitude."

He had more reservations. The objective of the meeting had changed. All the talk would be about the arrangement of personnel within the party after the return to Taiwan; it would be advisable not to get too involved in secret affairs like this, even though they all belonged to the same opposition party.

In the end, a compromise was reached. They would still attend the meeting, but after pleasantries had been exchanged, they would depart on a tour, using the rare chance of a visit to Europe as an excuse (nobody would have the heart to say no to a request from the Grieving National Mother to have a little fun); they would join a Taiwanese sightseeing group for a few days' tour, then return for the last two days of the meeting.

II

Why did she point out the man (whom she later learned was the devil) with the long, belt-like object tipped with an arrow that covered his private parts (which she later learned was a tail) to him when she saw the picture in the travel magazine?

They were on a tour bus at the time, heading toward another old town, another bridge, another church.

In addition to the group leader who traveled from Taiwan with them, the local guide assigned to the Taiwanese tour group was also an immigrant from Taiwan.

This guide was a slick, good-looking man. His face, originally handsome, had become lost in rolls of middle-aged fat, endowing him with a pair of drooping eyelids, a greasy nose, full lips, and a double chin.

Between quick introductions of place names, history, and famed sites, the guide told amusing stories nonstop, especially off-color jokes.

At first things were a bit awkward; quite a number of people in the group recognized her, and most of them felt sorry for her husband, locked up behind bars for all these years. While they didn't necessarily know of the nickname "Grieving National Mother" and wouldn't openly express their support for the political party she belonged to, no one who had any scant knowledge of her past had the heart to enjoy dirty jokes in front of her—a woman one might as well call a widow.

But the guide was hilarious; the sky outside the window was clearly blue as only the sky of a northern country where darkness doesn't fall till nine or ten in the evening could be blue; the river was a European river whose name no one could recall; the scenery was one of woods and hills covered in budding spring leaves, interspersed with small, red-gabled cottages—entirely different from the chaos and dust of the island they had come from.

And so, after the initial embarrassment, everyone joined in the boisterous laughter.

As for her, she'd heard descriptions of off-color jokes before (nobody would knowingly tell jokes like that in the presence of the Grieving National Mother) and more or less expected them to be grossly explicit; however, now that she had the chance to hear some first-hand, she discovered that most of them weren't all that easy to grasp: she often had trouble getting the gist of the jokes while everyone else on the bus roared with laughter.

She lifted the corners of her mouth though, and chimed in, her laugh gracious.

His response, on the other hand, was always instantaneous. In the beginning, because of her, his laughter was more or less stinted; however, after being immersed in the relaxed atmosphere of the group, he not only listened and laughed, but, like some other members, began telling dirty jokes of his own over the microphone during one particularly long drive.

Only he remained constantly aware of his status as opposition-party people's representative; his jokes, though bawdy, had political overtones (even politics can be converted into dirty jokes): "After communications opened up between our neighbor across the strait and us, a Taiwanese youth went to China and found himself a Chinese girlfriend, and soon after, they opened up three passages of communication."

Guffaws started in the audience.

"Having entered, the patriotic-minded Taiwanese thought, 'Now I've gone and poked a Chinese woman.' And so he quickly said, 'I have unified you.' 'Says who?' the Chinese woman retorted, 'Now I have Taiwan in my grip; only the two nut-size islands Jinmen and Matsu are left hanging outside.'"

She understood this joke, and began to laugh merrily, the peals of her laughter tinkling like strings of bells.

In all the years he'd known her, he had never heard her laugh like this.

The words "Grieving National Mother" first appeared in print in a tear-jerking article written by a pro-opposition party female writer.

In her story, she gave a moving sketch of the political prisoner's wife, by then a people's representative, whom she had run into by chance on a southbound train.

The ex-high school teacher who used to play the violin never wore anything but black business suits after she became a people's representative. She looked somber and unsure of herself at first; meanwhile, with the passage of time, the date of her husband's release seemed to recede farther and farther into the future.

She had thought that being a people's representative would at least endow her with some kind of status and lend her voice strength, which she hoped would be of help to her husband in his plight. Soon after her election into office, however, she came to realize that she was merely one out of the thousand or so people's representatives, and that, in an Assembly in which more than ninety percent of the members were under the autocrat's thumb, her voice wasn't just weak, it was inaudible —had she been able to make herself heard, it wouldn't have done any good anyway.

From then on, a mien of hopeless determination became a permanent part of her countenance. She calmly interrogated government officials in the Assembly, reading from her script word-for-word (which was of course written for her by her aides), intoning the sharpest possible questions about human life and human rights in her gentle, sorrowful voice. The effect was haunting.

The people who voted for her out of compassion never expected her to perform with such brilliance; all of a sudden, names like "Grieving National Mother" and "National Mother of Sorrow" flew thickly in the air.

The female writer wrote of how she expressed her admiration for the sacrifices the Grieving National Mother had made for the people, and also for her outstanding performance in the Assembly. But she, with her beautiful, eternally sad face against the blue velvet seat back of the southbound train, gazed into the distance out the window and said with infinite longing, "None of this is what I want; it means nothing to me at all. There is nothing great or admirable about me; I didn't choose to make these sacrifices willingly. All I want is to go back to the life I had before, with my husband back beside me, and a home of our own, and our two children."

She never shed a tear while saying all this; her eyes never even got moist. At the end, the writer wrote: "I shall never forget this wish of a wife and mother, which, despite its humbleness, may remain forever unfulfilled."

The dirty jokes on the bus continued, for not only did the guide, but also members of the tour, even the ladies, march up to the microphone to tell joke after joke; a matron some fifty years of age was a master hand at it.

The passengers' jokes were every bit as good as the guide's.

Without hints (he was naturally too embarrassed to explain these jokes, which involved mentioning organs by name and discussing sizes), she wasn't particularly interested in fathoming what made the jokes bawdy or why they were funny. Instead, she gave her attention to the scenery outside.

The bus had been following the river for some time when, rounding a sudden bend, it drove past a tiny isle, tens of meters from the bank, in the middle of the river. The isle was so small that only a lone white villa could fit on it; it was charmingly picturesque, standing in the middle of the emerald-green river like something out of a fairy tale. Before she could catch herself, she exclaimed out loud, "What is that?"

Hearing her, the guide glanced at the little isle with professional composure, saying easily, "Oh, I forgot to tell you folks, that's my house."

His tone was casual, but his voice boomed so strongly over the loud-speaker that it created the impression that he was speaking the irrefutable truth.

"Really?" Some people responded in unison.

"Sure. Please come to my humble dwelling for coffee at five tomorrow afternoon. Boats are at the wharf; there's one that leaves at four-thirty —you can catch that one or swim over, it's not that far."

For a moment, silence reigned on the bus. Then a male voice called, "Don't buy that crap!"

The guide began to chuckle, his laughter making smacking sounds over the loudspeaker as if he were blowing into the microphone.

"I've made this clear from the very start. What I say on this bus no longer counts once I get off it; if you come tomorrow it's your problem, I won't be held responsible."

Laughter and catcalls rippled through the passengers, then the guide's voice came on again, serious this time, "There's no way I could afford a place like that; it used to be the villa of a king, now it's a restaurant. I hear that they still keep their menu and their service fit for royalty, though."

The lighthearted irresponsibility of the guide seemed to open up new possibilities for those on the bus, for they shifted from telling dirty jokes to imitating the guide by making half-serious, half-joking promises and suggestions; most of the time it was difficult to distinguish between truth and bluff as people made fun of each other.

She turned toward him and, from the smile on her face, he thought she was going to tease him; but there was also a look of schoolgirl naiveté in her expression, an artless coquetry. Then he heard her say softly, "I read a lot of fairy tales when I was little and I almost came to believe the story of the Red Dancing Shoes. For a long time I refused to wear anything but red shoes. Regardless of how my family threatened and bribed, they couldn't get me to wear shoes of any other color. I always thought that if I kept on wearing red shoes, one of these days I would come across a pair that were the Red Dancing Shoes..."

The expression of delicate femininity on her face remained unchanged.

"I've never wanted anything in my life more than a house like the one on the river; I want to wear a long, full hoop-skirt, and come down the sweeping staircase to waltz in the great hall..."

"How undemocratic! Having such feudal ideas in an age like this—instead of 'Grieving National Mother,' we'd be better off calling you... calling you..." he was still in the joking mood and, without further thought, resumed teasingly, "'Cinderella's Godmother' will do; you're too old to be Cinderella..."

Then, realizing with a jolt that he'd never spoken to her in this manner before or used words like he had just used, he stopped.

Aside from his being a bright young church member who had had the courage to stand up for justice during the Reign of Terror, the greatest reason he had been elected people's representative was that he had been one of the Cannon's defense lawyers.

(Nobody would deny this, not even he. The defense attorney and the "martyr" were both symbols of that dark era, with the same halo around their heads.)

He wasn't even the chief lawyer representing the Cannon in court; the chief lawyer naturally became something bigger and better than a people's representative: he became a member of the Control Yuan. Our hero was only a paralegal in a law firm at the time; he lost his job because of his involvement in the attempted rescue of the Cannon, and became a member of the opposition.

During the next few years he became the chief editor of a magazine founded by the Cannon. (The magazine was prohibited time and again, as was to be expected, and had already gone through the names *Democrat*, *Forward*, *Autonomy*, *Progress*, *Prospect* and the like. Although it had to resurface with a new name after each banning, word still got around that this was the Cannon's magazine, and people continued to subscribe to it.)

This young editor with his flair for writing, his clear-mindedness (resulting from the training he'd received in law school), and his eloquence became the spokesperson of the new generation. Five of the most brilliant young people of the time came together to form an editors' alliance, masquerading as a consultant group for the magazine to avoid persecution from the regime. They became a new source of power among the dissenters and, several years later, in the officially acknowledged opposition party.

They were dubbed the "Corruption-Fighting Five," which was later shortened to "C-Fighting Five," and finally evolved into "Cougar-Fighting Five."

Nobody needed to be told who the "Cougar" was.

The people rallied for the man the brave little wife had recommended the same way they had rallied for her when she first ran for people's representative, voting him in to take her place in the Assembly after she'd moved ahead to become legislator.

And so, with her support, this paralegal with the gift for writing, this editor of pro-democratic magazines, this church-going member of the Cougar-Fighting Five entered the Assembly by a landslide victory.

The supply of lewd jokes must have eventually become exhausted, or perhaps they were simply no longer amusing; in any case, the guide began to talk about his womanizing experiences.

"Seriously, there's no woman a man can't get so long as he's brazen enough."

The usual titters rippled through the passengers.

"Sometimes you don't even have to say anything. I went to Madrid once, and to be honest, I knew practically no Spanish at all. So, I was sitting in this roadside cafe, and there was this girl sitting across from me—quite a chick she was! So I beckoned a waiter over, drew a cup of coffee on my napkin, and pointed to the girl. The waiter, comprehending, brought her a cup of coffee accordingly and pointed at me. The girl accepted, took a polite sip, and gave me a smile…"

The guide paused strategically, at which the passengers began to clamor, "What then? What then?"

"So I sat there a while longer, then asked for the waiter again. I drew a bed, on the napkin, and asked him to show it to the lady. Seeing that it was a bed, she simpered. I walked over to her then, and we went back to my hotel room together."

With the white villa on the isle fresh on their memories, it seemed that nobody was willing to believe him; it was a moment before somebody called from the rear, a woman's voice barely audible above the rumbling of the engine, "I don't believe it! Never heard of anyone bedding a girl by drawing a bed..."

"Take it or leave it," the guide's voice was strong over the loudspeaker, drowning everything else out. "The next morning she even taught me how to catch a local bus to the airport. It'd have cost me fifty bucks by taxi; it took only five by bus—saved me a lot of money, I'm telling you!"

"How could you communicate with her when you didn't speak Spanish?" the woman demanded.

"Oh come on, you still don't understand? What need is there for words in a situation like that? You just do the act."

Everyone sniggered.

"Well, to be serious, the young lady knew a little English, so I spoke some English and some German with her; and then we could also use gestures, and if all that wasn't good enough we could always draw."

"Yeah, right, you must be a really good artist," challenged the woman.

"Artist, my foot! I only know how to draw a camp cot."

At this, even the Grieving National Mother burst into laughter.

He couldn't remember ever having seen her laugh with such spontaneity before. He started to laugh along with everybody else, and then, without warning, a stab of infinite sadness pierced him through the heart.

It wasn't the Cannon's arrest that had permanently wiped the ready smile from her face. After the initial wracking despair, after the campaign for people's representative that saw her sobbing accusations through her tears from every rally podium, her life gradually settled into a kind of orderly resignation.

Though the haunting sadness never really left her face, she shed tears in public less and less frequently.

Especially after she became a legislator, and her approval ratings grew with her days in office (the information she needed for her interrogations came from sympathizers as well as through other channels, some from known sources, others from anonymous ones; to perform well she only had to make sure she did her homework), people almost came to discard her title of "Grieving National Mother" in exchange for "Brave National Mother."

If only she had not been separated from her two children.

Things immediately became extremely difficult for the two children, who at the time of their father's arrest were still in primary school.

The regime, with the media entirely under its control, propagated through broadcasts and printed matter alike that the people arrested were "violent," "treacherous," and "too evil to merit forgiveness." The children were tormented at school with names like "offspring of the convict" and "children of the felon" by schoolmates who had no way of knowing better.

Those who didn't join ranks with the rest didn't venture to openly give a helping hand either; only a very few teachers stood up to protect the children, using the slogans "education must be based on love" and "no discrimination among students" to justify their actions—for then nobody dared to say "politics shouldn't be involved in education."

For politics was education. In classes like Civil Education, some teachers reverently called the Big Arrest an act of justice for the upholding of morality.

The children were not only isolated, but turned into enemies of the country and the society.

Their mother tried to send them abroad, away from the country so mercilessly torturing them; permission to depart was of course denied, for the three of them were the best hostages the regime could find to make the Cannon behave, while he, locked up behind bars, was its surest pawn against them.

However, after a long struggle on the mother's part and, more significantly, with the combined efforts of overseas blacklisted members and international human rights organizations, the children finally got leave to depart for the United States (Fortunately for them their maternal grandparents resided there.).

It was then, after she lost her children, that the smile left the mother's face, more or less for good.

As he gazed upon her merry, glowing face, for one split second it seemed as if he had never seen this woman before.

It was at this moment that she pointed to the picture of a statue of a nude man in the travel magazine she had been leafing through, and inquired of him, "Who is this?"

"It's the devil," he replied without hesitation.

With his religious background he was naturally familiar with most of the figures within the Christian faith, and that enabled him to identify at a glance the horns on the head of the man in the picture and his arrow-tipped, pointed tail.

All that she noticed though was the handsome face of the statue and the cold, remote expression on it. The naked body was muscular, full of strength and beauty, yet there was a soft-looking belt wrapped round the lower part of the torso, creating a kind of conflict, striking a note of discord.

Once he had identified him as the devil for her, though, she saw that the two bumps among the thick, matted hair, though slight, were indeed horns, and the soft-looking belt-like thing tipped with the arrow was undeniably a pointed tail.

It wasn't till then that she realized that she had been pointing to the pointed tail hiding the loins of the devil statue, and asking a young man what it was. And that even the tail couldn't adequately cover the whole region; only with the aid of the thighs, bowed inwards ever so slightly, was total exposure avoided—yet what this achieved was more room for the imagination.

The blood rushed to her face then, flooding it a deep crimson.

III

She began to call him "Devil" in jest, because of the two horn-like tufts that often appeared on his head when he hadn't had the chance to comb his wavy hair, which he wore parted down the middle, after getting up in the mornings.

He led a veritable owl's life, retiring late each night and sleeping in every morning. As people's representative and magazine editor, there was always somebody he had to see and something he needed to discuss, and night was the time for social engagements in the city. The tour's scheduled morning calls at 7:00 a.m. often saw him at the breakfast table with his eyes bleary and his hair tousled.

He didn't always have two horns; sometimes the locks would all be to one side of his head so there was only one large horn, other times they stood up in clumps, creating three or four different ones. Most of the time though, he had two of them.

That was when she learned that he always washed his hair before sleeping each night, and that he often went to bed with his hair still damp so that it appeared in all sorts of curious shapes in the morning, depending on the position he slept in the night before.

(Sleeping on his side, long legs bowed slightly inward, it would help conceal...)

Since she called him "Devil," he retaliated by calling her "Cinderella's Godmother."

At first she had exclaimed indignantly, "Cinderella's Godmother? Am I that old?"

"Do you really think you can be Cinderella still?" he quipped.

Stunned, she made no reply.

So he called her that, "Cinderella's Godmother," which eventually got shortened to "Godmother" (sometimes said in English). It took him a while to realize that she disliked being called "Godmother" so intensely because she wasn't fond of the word "mother."

In some ways, she'd stopped maturing after the night of the Big Arrest.

She'd just turned thirty-two the Christmas of the Big Arrest. She was a high school music teacher who practiced Japanese tea-making and flower-arranging and who loved to read literature. She belonged to a generation of women who grew up watching movies like *The Great Waltzes*, in which characters floated down the sweeping staircase in a trailing hoop-skirt to waltz with a man in a carnival mask and black tuxedo in a marble hall lighted with a crystal chandelier...

She lost her husband in the Big Arrest, and thus lost her love, her sex life, and her marriage. She knew she could be nothing but the Grieving National Mother thenceforth, and would only be able to live through the upcoming days and nights as such.

She lived through the worst traumas of life, and learned of the coldness of reality through politics; in those aspects she grew at manifold the speed of other women her age. In the world of love, though, her growth had frozen to a standstill. She never got the chance to grow weary of married life, or tire of being a wife, or watch her own youth fade while playing the role of mother through the years.

Her romance and her love life as a woman had forever ceased to be in her thirty-second year, on the Christmas Eve of the Big Arrest.

She wasn't the only person setting limits to her actions; none of the people around her would have encouraged her otherwise. The Cannon was suffering in prison for the people, and she, as his wife, should certainly be true to his noble ideal. Besides, the Grieving National Mother anchored the resources and the morale of the opposition camp; even the slightest hint of a love affair on her part would inevitably be blown up into a scandal that would lead to fewer seats for her party in the Legislature, the Assembly, and the provincial parliaments.

And so they put up with her almost uncontrollable mood swings, which seemed dependent on the monthly cycle of the moon. In spite of prescriptions from the doctor to mitigate the magnitude of her fluctuations as well as her own best efforts to suppress them, neither appeared to be doing much good.

As editor of the magazine (after some twenty bannings and confiscations, it was currently named *Overcome*), he was one of the most important of her aides; not only did he analyze the pros and cons of any given action and deduce political maneuvers for her, but he was also the person who knew how to best handle her.

This bright young opposition party people's representative, reputed for his cutting, merciless pen, had the sensitivity that often went with a talent for words. To her closest assistants he said, "Treat her the way you would a young girl. Soothe her, pamper her a little."

It was springtime in Europe, and late in the season already, with lilacs fragrant, peonies bright, tulips blooming, azaleas covering the bushes, and pansies and sops-in-wine thickly carpeting the ground.

Except there were no roses yet.

Through the sea of flowers they came to a forlorn castle. Built in the eleventh century, it had looming ramparts of limestone with narrow windows set high in them; closed and confining, it was very different from the bright, ornate palaces of later ages.

They started out animatedly recounting stories of their youth along the way; and after she began teasingly calling him "Devil" it was as though she'd freed him from a spell: he reverted to the way most thirty-year-olds of his generation talked—cutting and merciless, sarcastic to the extreme, yet intensely amusing. He often left her speechless with indignation, yet unable to stop laughing. She was entirely incapable of defending herself against his bantering, so all she could do was raise her small fists and hit him with them.

Occasionally, when she truly felt offended, she would pull a long face. And he, picking up on this, would try to cajole her back into her former good humor with all sorts of compliments, his tone always bantering so that it was impossible to tell whether he meant what he said or not. And she, never really mad at him anyway, would be in kinks of laughter again before long.

Strolling through the old castle they saw high walls and tiny windows all around; the floor was of bare cobblestones, the limestone walls were void of all decoration. Dim and oppressive, the barrenness seemed to be under the power of some sinister spell, as if there were numberless ghosts from ages past imprisoned there, waiting to be set free.

"This looks so much like Dracula's castle," he remarked.

"Yeah, and you, the Devil, can be a part-time vampire," she teased, mimicking his way of speech.

"Oh no, I'm the vampire's pig."

She chuckled merrily. "Oh really, I never knew that the vampire had a pig before!"

"Of course a Taiwanese vampire has to have a pig! That way it'll have pig's blood soup and pig's blood cake to eat anytime it wants."

Laughingly, she pummeled him with her fists, her peals of mirth so weakening her that she practically had to lean against him. Putting an arm around her shoulders, he said, "I finally know what to call you now. You're 'Sleeping Beauty's Godmother.' This Godmother has fallen into deep slumber like Sleeping Beauty, and has not wakened since."

"So who's going to rouse Sleeping Beauty's Godmother, then?" she asked.

"Who do you think?" he countered.

(Since when did he start talking about anything other than politics anyway?)

Somebody was playing the fiddle in the restaurant, a middle-aged man with dark skin, either of Gypsy or South European origin (they couldn't tell which). His deep-set, dark eyes squinted as he fiddled, gazing directly, hypnotically with wistful sentimentality into whichever pair of eyes his happened to meet. But that sentimentality, achieved too effortlessly and displayed once too often, made the not entirely black eyes look unexpectedly chilly.

All the tunes he played were songs from the sixties and the seventies (the restaurant was for the most part filled up with tourists ranging from middle-aged to elderly), and most of them were American songs ("Unchained Melody," "You've Lost That Loving Feeling," "Do That to Me One More Time").

And he played the waltz.

There was somebody selling flowers in the restaurant, a cool-looking young Caucasian girl. Probably on account of the warmth of the spring, she wore a dress with a revealingly low neckline and billowing skirts. After seeing a lady holding a bunch of white lilacs walk by, he summoned the girl with the small basket.

The girl took a bunch of lilies of the valley from her basket, a spray of delicate white blossoms the locals called "little bells of May."

He bought two bunches.

Although she'd already known that the flowers were for her, she still felt her eyes brimming with tears (How long had it been since she had last felt warm tears in her eyes? With the glistening drops in them, her eyes were no longer cold, no longer full of heartbreak.). As she took the flowers in her hands she caught a whiff of their heavy perfume and exclaimed, astonished, "Oh, I didn't know they had flowers as fragrant as these in the northern lands." She sounded a little flustered, "Sweet-smelling flowers don't just grow in Taiwan... jasmines and gardenias and banana magnolias and... and... oh, what else is there?"

He watched her silently.

That night, the lilies of the valley lay nestled against her chest, pinned to the low neck of her nightgown. The flower stalks weren't long, a mere six or seven centimeters; the white blossoms held their wee mouths open like many tiny little bells, exuding cloud upon cloud of sweet fragrance.

The fragrance was in fact disturbing her sleep.

(Rumpled hair standing up in one clump, or several, gave off a faint smell of flowers. The last few days it'd smelled of spring meadows, and she, discovering that it came from the hotel's complimentary shampoo, began using it too, so that after a couple days she seemed to be immersed in the smell of him from head to toe.

She recommended using her moisturizing lotion. With the low humidity of the European climate being so different from the damp warmth of the island, his lips were chapped and his cheeks dry and tingling. He agreed to try the lotion, but could not be induced to use her lip balm, deeming that it was too feminine.

So he, too, smelled of her, or perhaps it would be better to say that they had the same smell because they breathed the same scents. Unlike her, though, his scent could only be detected from up close. From afar, he simply smelled clean, a combination of soap, shampoo, and a trace of facial cream.)

The lilies of the valley opened their little mouths as though specifically for the purpose of pouring forth their fragrance; the heavy perfume flowed from each little opening, not in ripples or waves, but in a swamping tide, leaving her feeling slightly suffocated.

The fragrance was in fact disturbing her sleep.

She could feel the lilies of the valley melting warm against her chest through the long night.

The lilies of the valley with their long, thick leaves. The flowers and green leaves resting in the valley between her breasts. They seemed to nestle closer to her fiery, beating heart when she lay down and her breasts flattened. The white bells, like little mouths with parted lips, suckled her bare skin, cool at first. And, awaiting fulfillment, the little openings formed by the petals grew warm and moist against her pulsating heart.

The bells were white and full of heat. And when the accommodating little mouths grew weary of holding themselves open, the edges, wilting, curled up slightly. The wide green leaves were as stiff as ever; through the fine silk of the nightgown they lay in the vee between her breasts (lying down with her breasts flattened, they pressed even closer against her body), and when she stirred they caressed her breasts, their tips brushing against her nipples. The leaves continued to tease her nipples (it was even a little bit painful, the leaves being as firm and hard as they were), and the nipples, notwithstanding, slowly grew taut (what if the leaves were touching some other part of her body?).

So she had to lie in one position, perfectly still. Even so, she couldn't stay in any one position she preferred but had to lie flat on her back to avoid crushing the spray of little white flowers against her chest. And lying thus, the bunch of flowers and leaves, close to ten centimeters in length (they seemed to have grown longer), bore down upon her breasts with their slight weight, pressing against her—especially since they were nestling there in the valley between her breasts.

The flowers were in truth disturbing her sleep.

(Sleeping on his side, long legs bowed slightly inward, it would help conceal...)

The arrow was in that particular place; she couldn't have been entirely unaware of the fact. When she had pointed there, the knowledge must have been lurking somewhere in her subconsciousness.

But the arrow was so extraordinary. When she placed her finger on the page and kept it centered there, wondering, "Why is there something like this here?"

If the tail hadn't been curving horizontally around the torso, if the tip of the triangular arrow hadn't been pointing sideways, but had stood vertically with the arrow aiming upwards, or if it had hung down toward the ground, it would have been easy to comprehend that the arrow was merely a symbol for something else.

However, with the arrow on its side, she was no longer certain what it was, and that was why she had to point at it and ask him. Was she only inquiring about the arrow, though? About the tail?

Sleeping on his side, long legs bowed slightly inward, it would help conceal... Or perhaps because of the angle his body was at—tilted to one side—the triangular arrow would really point sideways then; and if so, the pointed tail would of course be horizontal to his body also.

The flowers were in truth disturbing her sleep.

The moment she turned onto her side the little white lilies of the valley and the long leaves pinned to her front all swung sideways, making it extremely easy to bend or break them, so she had to reach up and gently prod the nosegay back into position, either letting it remain upright or hang upside-down.

When the morning light slanted into the room, the little bells, having been steeped in the raging, molten heat of her body all night long, seemed to have melted and secreted a thick, sticky substance that filled the little mouths formed by the petals so that they could no longer open to pour forth wave upon wave of perfume. Thus they fell into eternal slumber, never to wake again.

And the long, thick leaves, having been pressed against her feverish body the whole night, were no longer stiff in the morning. Soft and wilted, the edges were straight no more, neither were the tips sharp and piercing.

It was the end of their holiday.

They had come to this old city in Europe to attend a no-longer-secret gathering of blacklisted people. She was a legislator from the island. He was a people's representative.

The name of the meeting, Return of the Salmon, was inspired by the spirit of the fish, which, swimming upstream through countless obstacles, returns home to die in its birthplace. The exiles had been determined to challenge the ban upon the blacklist—with their lives if necessary— to win the right after thirty or more years abroad to set foot upon their native soil once more.

They usually had a banquet with traditional Taiwanese dishes at meetings like this: fried rice noodles, meat potage, rice cakes, and pork-stew-topped-rice were a must. And they would sing "Homeland in the Dusk" over and over again, their eyes full of tears, their sorrow boundless.

Although the tune was Japanese, the translated lyrics eloquently expressed the nostalgia of wandering sons and daughters for their fatherland. Nothing befitted gatherings like this better than a Japanese melody tinged with sadness—the topic of discussion would invariably come around to how the regime from China had proven to be tenfold more brutal to the Taiwanese than had their Japanese predecessors, foreign conquerors though they were.

All these were necessary proceedings at gatherings like this.

After the death of the dictator, however, the blacklist began to disintegrate. The tragic beauty of the salmon's homecoming was a thing of the past, and the meeting, planned for over the course of a year, turned into a get-together at which activities to be held after the return to Taiwan were mapped out.

Therefore her presence at the meeting no longer held symbolic meaning —the union of victims of the regime from the island and from abroad —but she insisted on coming; the official reason she gave was: "Just to show my gratitude."

However, those closest to her knew that her decision had been affected by her husband.

After the dictator's death, the ban on the blacklist wasn't the only thing that fell apart: all the Big Arrest prisoners, locked up for close to ten years, were suddenly in line for parole, edging closer to freedom with each passing day. Most of them eagerly awaited the termination of their unjust imprisonment, so they could be free to resume their posts in the struggle for democratic reform.

Only the Cannon, with characteristic doggedness, steadfastly maintained his innocence: he would not accept a parole for a crime he never committed; the only way to make him leave his cell was to publicly acknowledge his innocence.

Despite the death of its leader, the autocracy remained firmly rooted; there was no chance of the Cannon's demand being met. What it meant then was that he would stay in prison after his former comrades-in-arms had all been set free.

Allegedly the wife, hearing of her husband's decision during one of her visits, was unable to hide her tears. The only comment she ever made was, "You've never once thought about me all these years."

After that, she stuck fast to her decision to make the journey to Europe.

She agreed to play "Homeland in the Dusk" on the violin at the farewell party.

The party would mark the end of exile and suffering for these Taiwanese people. Hopefully during future meetings there would be no more need to sing with tears in their eyes,

Calling to me, calling to me,

My homeland is summoning me through the dusk.

Beckoning for my weary body to return,

This wanderer; this migrating bird without a home.

The party celebrated the end of sorrow and a joyous new beginning.

She needed a violin and a formal gown. She had nothing in her luggage but her business suits, and on an occasion like this—an important moment of bittersweet rejoicing—even she was unwilling to wear a suit while she played the violin.

Like the spouses of most overseas dissenters, the European chair's wife often had to organize Taiwanese banquets for twenty or thirty people at a moment's notice; coming up with a gown that would fit the Grieving National Mother was therefore all in a day's work for her.

The gown, like most evening wear for spring and summer, left the back and shoulders tantalizingly bare.

The ladies all agreed that exposing this much of her back and shoulders was required by etiquette in Europe. (Perhaps they had been away from Taiwan for so long that they failed to realize there were no sleeveless items in her wardrobe. Perhaps they, banned from the island for thirty or forty years, had no way of knowing that she rarely wore colors other than black, navy, or white.)

Nevertheless, gazing upon her own gowned reflection in the full-length mirror, she made no objection.

So what he saw in the soft glow of the lamps was the slender figure of a woman in a gown of dark wine. Her thinness belied her true age:

the long hair, swept up, revealed the graceful curve of her neck; the exposed shoulders and chest showed her fine bones. And where bare neck, shoulder, and arm came together—there rested the honey-colored violin.

The sleek, gleaming violin, its curves luscious and smooth, perched lightly on the expanse of creamy skin like the reclining figure of a woman. (Her neck and shoulders were a paler color. There would be tiny hairs on the back of her neck, and they would coyly bow to the lightest breath against her.)

The smooth, cold instrument, seemingly fragile, had a certain hardness to it; the end, firmly tucked between jaw and shoulder, fit against the curve of her neck. Her soft flesh and satiny skin cushioned the hard wood against her bones, so that the two met in a kiss that left eternal marks upon the contours of her body in his memory.

And the cold instrument, nestling against the heat of her body, slowly grew warm, for, resting where hills rose and valleys dipped over her fiery heart, it awaited the final burst of passion and flame.

The lusciously curved instrument would finally merge into one with the female body.

Just as the bow rose and the music swelled, he saw, albeit for one fleeting moment, the naked flesh of a woman standing amidst dreamlike light and shadow upon a stage not far away.

(And accompanying her like a shadow, the reclining body of the violin —gleaming, silken, curvaceous, awaited the fall of the bow.)

And fall the bow would—the long, slim bow. Falling upon the strings of the violin the way a dragonfly flits across water, or pressing closely against them, manipulating the violin to song. The repeated thrusts of the bow, penetrating and withdrawing by turns, and the monosyllabic cries merged into one continuous flow of music, becoming, with the motion of the bow, an eternal melody passed down through the generations.

But she had to complete this everlasting melody on her own. She had to hold the bow herself, and put it to the curvy violin resting against her shoulder: she had to press the bow onto the waiting strings to make music—alone. The strokes of the bow, guided by her hand, melded into one continuous flow of music.

In that split second, with the bow falling and the music on the verge of bursting forth, he saw strings of sparkling teardrops fall.

Once more, they stepped onto the bridge.

They were again staying in the hotel fronting the river. Her room still faced the bridge linking the two banks of the august city, the one famed for the statues lining it; his still faced the other way.

This would be their last night in the hotel by the bridge.

The last meeting had come to a perfect ending, after which they had a difficult time dissuading the chairman of the European section from keeping them company. She had said she would like to look around the city once more, for there were too many memories here worth cherishing for the rest of her life.

Without further comment he had fallen into step beside her, and they began to walk in the direction of the bridge.

"Most of these overseas people have never really done anything. Unlike exiles from some other countries, they never resorted to violence, bombs, and assassinations. All the same, they've been barred from their homeland for thirty, maybe forty years," he mused, still under the spell of the meeting earlier on. She nodded silently, but it was obvious she didn't care much for topics like this.

"For decades, they've been charged with the most preposterous accusations, and now, just because somebody died and things have started to open up, these accusations are suddenly dropped and they can go home again—just like that." He went on, "Frankly, it frightens me."

"Why?" Her concern for him showed.

"If things continue like this, Taiwan will become more and more democratic; I'm afraid that when that happens we won't know where we are at any longer."

"Wouldn't that be better? I wouldn't be a legislator anymore, and you wouldn't be a people's representative; we..."

She never finished what she was going to say.

"I am afraid we will soon discover that everything is in the process of falling apart, and past sacrifices will become unnecessary—meaningless even. When the new age comes, you, and all these people overseas, your sacrifices..."

She reached out, took his hand and said, quietly and firmly, "Look, the bridge."

The summer sun still lingered in the sky, and vendors, entertainers, and tourists crowded the bridge. Street musicians sang American love songs to the accompaniment of simple folk instruments; some trio or quartet performed a harmony.

They wove through the crowd to the music. The old man selling marionettes had a whole rack full of colorful, elaborately designed puppets: a long-nosed witch; a pot-bellied, one-eyed brigand with a bushy beard; a wild woman with flowers and grass scattered among her flaming hair that fell nearly to her knees.

She suggested taking pictures on the bridge. She had the rack full of puppets for her backdrop, while he chose a nearby statue for his. Holding the camera, she watched him approach the figure, and then, quite suddenly, she heard his astonished exclamation, "Why, isn't this the sculpture of the devil!"

Putting down the camera she came up to him, and there it was, the statue in the travel magazine, standing as large as life before her.

The devil had now become a three-dimensional reality, tall and looming, the stone gray-green from the ravages of time, the edges dulled. But there really were horns in the wild hair, the handsome face was still coldly immobile, and the tail, curling from his back to the center of his lower body, ended in a triangular arrow.

The life-sized statue afforded a clearer view, and now she noticed that the arrow on the tip of the tail wasn't big; still it amply concealed the vital part on his lower body, leaving the area flat. Obviously he read her thoughts, for he said with a hint of playfulness, "Only statues of heroic figures are allowed to accentuate that part, you know, so that's off-limits for devils. Long ago at church we used to joke about how every devil sculpture wears a tight, invisible jockstrap that completely hides and suppresses the important part."

Glancing toward the sculpture, he continued wickedly, "Look! This devil is wearing more than a jockstrap—it has a chastity belt on! Everything is…"

"A devil with a chastity belt?" Her words, though hesitant, cut him short.

"Sure enough! A devil with a chastity belt—now fancy that, what more is there left for a devil to do when he has a chastity belt on?"

His bantering tone faded as the ambiguity of his unintentional pun dawned on him; his voice grew brittle, and abruptly stopped.

IV

Were the pro-opposition female writer to narrate these events, she might write something to this effect: Who, really, is the Devil in the chastity belt? He, or she?

  * From *Pa-shih-su-nien tua-pien-shao-shuo-hsiun* 《八十四年短篇小說選》 (*Annual Anthology of Short Stories, 1995*), ed. Liao Hsien-hao (Taipei: Elite Publishing Co., 1996). This translation won the eleventh Liang Shih-chiu Literary Award for Translation.

Chapter 11

The Fish

大青魚

Chen Jo-hsi 陳若曦

(Translated by Nancy C. Ing 殷張蘭熙)

Foreman K'uai came home early today. As soon as he pushed open the door, he popped in his head and asked his wife, who was lying in bed, "How are you feeling? Any better?"

At the sound of the door opening, Mama K'uai had turned her head, and, seeing it was her husband, her face lit up with unexpected pleasure. She didn't want to worry him so she answered evasively, "Seems better. Doesn't hurt so much."

It was the end of February and still bitterly cold. The windows and doors were tightly shut with wads of newspaper stuffed into the cracks. The smell of Chinese herbal medicine permeated the room.

"Have you taken your medicine?" Foreman K'uai glanced at the earthen pot on the small round table beside the bed.

"Yes, Sister Chang got it ready. She even cooked lunch for me."

Although the person who had done all this was not present, Mama K'uai's voice was filled with gratitude. Her old backaches had come back, and for the past few days she had been in bed most of the time. Had it not been for the neighbors' help, Foreman K'uai would have been unable to go to work.

"How come you're home so early today?" she asked with a glance at the old clock hanging on the wall near the foot of the bed. It was only three.

Foreman K'uai worked at the dockyards with two apprentices, and his work and meetings kept him busy from morning to night. His home was quite some distance away, so he had to change buses to reach Cock Crow Temple from Yangtze River Bridge, and he never got home before dark.

"This afternoon we were supposed to have political study. But they said some American newspaper reporters were coming to Nanking, so at the last minute it was changed to a general cleanup. My two apprentices are really thoughtful. They know you're at home sick and they wouldn't let me do anything. They practically forced me to come back."

As he talked, the old man took off his gloves, poured himself a glass of hot water from the thermos bottle on top of the chest of drawers, and cupped his hands around the glass for warmth.

When she heard this, Mama K'uai smiled. "These two young fellows seem to be all right. Let's just hope they won't be like the last ones, who turned against you as soon as the Cultural Revolution began, and cursed you like you weren't worth a cent!"

The old man's lips broadened into a grin as he sat down by the small round table. He blew on the glass of hot water before taking a tentative sip; then, finding that it was not too hot, he gulped it all down.

"What else could they do under the circumstances?" he said without resentment. "The campaign was in full swing and they had to take a radical stand; they did not want to get into trouble themselves. They were sorry afterward and used to come to me when no one was around and apologize for what they did. At the time their only thought was the revolution, neglecting their work entirely. Now whenever they come up against any difficulty, don't they always come running to me?"

"That's because you're too good-hearted!"

Mama K'uai laughed. She was able to accept the incident now and take it in stride. But two years before, when she learned that the old man's apprentice had attacked him in bulletin-board posters, she had really been upset. She was especially disturbed by the fiasco when she invited the apprentice for New Year's Eve dinner one year. It had been entirely her idea, but the apprentice had accused the old man of having ulterior motives. The old man was said to be going the way of the imperialists, trying to "cultivate" and "corrupt" young workers. He had been forced up onto the stage for confession and self-criticism. The old woman had seethed with anger.

"Speaking of my apprentices, I almost forgot!" the old man exclaimed. "They say that during the welcome for the American reporters, the markets will be better stocked than usual the next couple of days, especially the market on Tung Jen Street. They said you can get anything you want. Tell me what you'd like to eat and I'll go out and get it for you."

The old woman closed her eyes and thought it over. She had not been to market for over a week. The old man had to pick up what he could on his way home after work, with the result that he had brought back nothing but cabbage that had been frozen. It had been cabbage with soy sauce one day and cabbage with salt pork the next. As the old woman had a bad stomach anyway, the monotony of the diet had robbed her of what little appetite she ever had.

"I just want a taste of fish soup," the old woman said, her eyes brightening at the prospect. "It would be nice if you could get a fish! You can cook it with a few slices of ginger, some scallions, and a dash of rice wine when the soup is done. Ah, that would be delicious!"

Hearing this description, the old man's mouth began to water.

"Eat fish? All right, you can count on it!"

He stood up and straightened out the cotton-padded hat that he had not taken off his head, then patted the pocket of his quilted jacket to make sure his money was there.

"I'll go to the Tung Jen Street market right away. My young fellows say they've got everything there!"

He went into the kitchen, looked in at the stove, and was pleased to see a circle of blue flame underneath. He opened the bottom door a slit wider to get a little more ventilation before picking up the market basket. Considering the distance between Cock Crow Temple and Tung Jen Street, he decided to go by bicycle. As the bicycle was stored under the bed, it took him some time to get it out. The tires were flat, of course, so he had to go and find the air pump to pump them up again. After all this effort, the old man was breathing hard, but when he thought of the fish that he was going to buy, he felt elated. The old woman watched him bustling about, and thought of the fish that he was going to bring home, her face also filled with pleasure.

"I'm leaving," he called out as he pushed his bicycle out the door.

"Come back early," responded the old woman. "Just as long as you buy a fish, it'll be all right."

As soon as he turned out of the small lane, he was on Cock Crow Temple Road, which led all the way to the south gate of People's Park and was always crowded. Being accustomed as he was to lining up for the bus in the darkness of early dawn, the bicycle gave him a sense of freedom and exhilaration. As he wove right and left among the pedestrians, the hoarse sound of the bell whenever he pressed it sounded pleasant to him. When he turned onto Peking Avenue, the road became wider and there was more traffic. One after another, trucks whizzed past him, speeding toward Drum Tower Circle. The old man had always dreaded the traffic at the circle, so he turned off onto a small alley and, taking a short cut, quickly reached Tung Jen Street.

It had been a long time since he had visited the market. The last time was over a year ago when his son had come back on home leave from the Northeast, and he had gotten up especially early in the morning to buy a chicken.

The market on Tung Jen Street and the Central Market on New Market Square were both well known. The City Revolutionary Committee looked upon them as places of importance, so they were excellently managed and always well stocked with a wide assortment of fish, meat, and vegetables. Although many people came from far away to shop here, the K'uai family did not usually come here to buy its food. First of all, they did not live nearby. Second, most of the people who patronized these two markets were the Liberation Army people and the servants for the families of high-level party members who lived around that area. They spent money quite freely, and Mama K'uai, who had been frugal all her life, disapproved of their ways.

Foreman K'uai saw that since his last visit the entire street had been renovated. The street had been swept clean and the walls carefully washed; the newly posted political slogans were particularly eye-catching. Whether they were selling soy sauce, pickled vegetables, groceries, brooms, or toilet paper, the shops on both sides of the street looked as if they had all been carefully rearranged. The glass windows were gleaming with cleanliness, and even the entries had been so well scrubbed that the bricks displayed a vivid red.

At the entrance to the marketplace, he parked his bicycle, picked up his basket, and walked in. Upon entering, he saw that the cement floor had just been washed so that not a speck of dirt could be seen. As he walked, Foreman K'uai could not help but look back at the footprints made by his large, cotton-padded shoes. This made him feel somewhat guilty. There were not too many customers in the market but every stall had some business. Each seller wore a knee-length apron that had been washed and starched a snowy white, while those selling meat and fish even had white cotton hats on their heads. Since his mind was on the fish for his wife, he passed by the stall selling pork and made his way toward the fish stall.

Of all the stalls in this market, he most admired the fish stall. The counter was built of shiny tiles, which made the various kinds of fish laid out on display appear even more appealing to the eye. From far away, he could see the ribbon-fish and bream that covered the stand. There was already a line waiting. As he was about to hurry over to join the line, he suddenly saw there were other fish behind the counter. He stepped forward to look. There were indeed four or five large ch'ing-yu displayed in a row, their bodies shining and looking very fresh.

Why buy bream when there is ch'ing-yu? he thought. Bream had a muddy taste that no amount of seasoning could get rid of.

He saw a seller busily weighing fish, calling out the weights while his free hand clicked the abacus. Another man squatted in a corner sorting fish from a large wooden box, throwing the large ones into one basket and the small ones into another.

Old K'uai wanted to catch the attention of the man who was sorting fish, so he called out, "Are these ch'ing-yu for sale?"

The seller looked up, frowning at him for some time before he answered. "They're out on the stand, so of course they're for sale."

"Then weigh half a fish for me!"

As he spoke, he placed his basket beside the stand, thinking fast as to which half of the fish he should buy. Mama K'uai had said she wanted to have fish soup, and the fish head would make an even tastier soup than a chicken! He had better buy the top half.

Having made up his mind, he said to the man, "Give me the top half with the head."

"Can't sell half a fish," the seller answered, shaking his head as he went back to his sorting without another look at the old man. "If you want it, you'll have to take the whole fish!"

The old man hesitated. Buy the whole fish? He looked at the price mark —sixty-five cents a catty. One whole fish would come to two or three dollars. His hand instinctively moved up to the pocket of his quilted jacket.

"Well?" the seller asked, raising his head again. Seeing the other's indecision, he added coldly, "Each weighs about four or five catties."

K'uai was annoyed by the man's attitude. He patted the top part of his jacket where this month's pay, which he had just received, lay hidden in his inner pocket.

"Okay, go ahead and weigh the whole fish!" he answered briskly.

The fish seller seemed taken aback. Giving the old man a hard look, he slowly got up and walked over. Without a word, he picked up a large fish and put it on the hook of the scale's steelyard.

"Oh, take that one." K'uai hastily pointed to a smaller fish.

"What's the matter?" The seller pretended not to understand. Lifting the steelyard higher, he swung the dangling fish in front of his customer's face and the fish's tail nearly brushed against K'uai's chin.

The old man took a step backward and waved his hand in a conciliatory gesture. "Go ahead, weigh it." He'd better not make a fuss over it, he decided. He consoled himself with the thought that it was a rare opportunity to get such good fish, though it meant they would have to eat fish for the next three days. Luckily the weather was still cold and the fish would not spoil.

"Sixty-five cents, four catties and a half make it two dollars, ninety-three cents!" The salesman blinked his eyes and announced without bothering to use the abacus.

Hurriedly the old man took out a five-dollar note from his inner pocket. The seller took it, gave him his change, and carefully placed the fish in the basket. After another curious look at the old man, he went back to sorting fish.

K'uai let out a deep sigh. He picked up his basket and left the fish stall with a feeling of satisfaction. *Those young fellows were right,* he thought. *This Tung Jen Street market was quite a place; one could actually buy such a large ch'ing-yu here. My wife won't believe her eyes when she sees the size of this fish!*

Wrapped in his own contentment, his mouth curled up into a happy grin, he did not notice the curious looks he got from the other customers, some of whom even pointed at his basket.

As he passed by a vegetable stand, K'uai's eyes lit up. The end of February was always a time when produce was scarce, and he would never have thought that there could be so many kinds of vegetables on display. In addition to the turnips, carrots, and frozen cabbages usually available, there were also tomatoes and cucumbers, which he had not seen for a long time. These delicacies were attractively displayed in separate little baskets placed at the most prominent spots in the stand. He looked at the price mark of the tomatoes—fifty cents a catty. He could only shake his head. *They were purposely priced too high for people to buy,* he thought. In the summer they were only five cents a catty. There was no price mark on the cucumbers. *His wife had always been fond of cucumbers,* he reflected, *and he would get one for whatever the price, just so that she could taste something fresh. Having been in for so many days, she would enjoy the taste of something different.*

"How much are the cucumbers?" he asked a woman vender.

"The cucumbers are not for sale!" she answered bluntly, her eyes fixed on the fish in his basket.

The old man was disappointed, but there was nothing he could do, so he looked around to see what he could get to cook with the fish head.

"Hurry! Hurry! There are people waiting behind you!" The woman gestured impatiently with the steelyard, sending the lead weight and bronze plate of the scale clanging against each other.

Being hurried, K'uai became flustered, unable to make up his mind. All of a sudden he remembered that they might not have any ginger at home. "Give me half a catty of tender ginger."

Just then he spotted a small basket of bamboo shoots in a corner. He knew that bamboo shoots were very expensive, but they would be delicious cooked with the fish head. He thought of how frugal his wife had been through the years. Now that she was ill, she deserved at least one good meal. Bamboo shoots cooked with fish head... he had not indulged in such luxury in years.

"Give me two bamboo shoots." This time he did not even bother to ask the price.

"Sixty-five cents a catty," the woman announced. She emptied the ginger into his basket and went over to weigh the bamboo shoots.

After he paid for the bamboo shoots he picked up the basket, and, feeling its weight, decided not to buy anything more, but to go straight home to cook the fish. There were countless varieties of dishes displayed in the glass showcases on the prepared food counter, but he gave them only a cursory glance as he hurried toward the main gate.

More people were coming to shop now—housewives, laborers coming from work, political cadres, and soldiers in neat uniforms were pouring into the market.

He walked over to where he had parked his bicycle. There were now more bicycles alongside his own.

"Comrade, is there any more of that fish left?" A man who had brushed by him had turned back to ask anxiously.

"Yes!" he assured the man enthusiastically. "Hurry, there are still several—"

Before he had finished speaking, a housewife carrying a basket hurried up to him and broke in: "Comrade, how much is this fish selling for? Is there a long waiting line?"

"Not long really. Sixty-five cents a catty."

Seeing that his basket had attracted so much attention, K'uai took another look at the large ch'ing-yu curled up in the basket. With its clear bulging eyes and bright scales, it was a very impressive-looking fish indeed. The old man's heart was filled with a pleasant feeling.

He carefully hung the basket on the handlebar of his bicycle. Because of the crowd, he pushed his bicycle along and walked out to Tung Jen Street. At the entrance, just as he was about to get on his bicycle, someone tapped him on the shoulder.

"Hey, comrade, take that fish back."

The old foreman lowered his right leg to the ground. He turned and saw a middle-aged man with small protruding eyes. From his manner and dress, the old man could tell he was a political cadre.

"What did you say?" K'uai thought the man had mistaken him for someone else.

"The fish isn't for sale," the man said in a low voice, trying to be patient. "You take it back to the cashier's office immediately. They'll give you back what you paid for it."

"What?" Hearing this, the old man quickly raised his voice. "Not for sale? Damn it! Then why the hell didn't they say so in the first place? Now you snatch it away when it is about to be dropped into the pot!"

Hearing the old man's curse, the cadre's face hardened and his eyes glared.

"If they're all sold out, what'll be left to show the foreign visitors when they arrive?"

The old man had wanted to say something more to give vent to his grievance, but when he heard the words "foreign visitors," he stopped short. With the mention of foreign visitors the issue was closed. He gulped and blinked his eyes in stony silence.

The cadre, seeing that he was silent, demanded menacingly, "What unit do you belong to?"

Foreman K'uai became angry at the insolent tone of voice and blurted out, "Nanking Dockyard, iron worker for thirty years!" To save himself from further questioning, K'uai gave his type of work and the length of time he had served.

Hearing that he was an old worker, the cadre softened and nodded his head. "Nevermind; you didn't know. Just take the fish back. The cashier's office will—"

The old foreman broke in, "If you want the fish, you take it! I won't!"

K'uai remembered the hard looks he had gotten from that fish seller. If he took this fish back, not only the seller, but all the people in the market would stare at him.

By that time several people had gathered around, looking curiously at the two men. The cadre was afraid the matter might get out of hand, so he backed down and said, "I'll take it back for you. You wait here; I'll bring the money back to you right away."

Without waiting for an answer, he hurriedly reached into the basket and grabbed the fish. With his hand hooked in the gill of the fish and every eye riveted on him, he walked toward the back gate of the marketplace.

K'uai looked on helplessly as the fish, its huge tail swinging back and forth, disappeared into the distance. He looked into his basket again. Except for two pieces of ginger root and two withered bamboo shoots, it was empty. He could go back and try to buy a bream, but it would probably be all sold out by now. Then, thinking of the long waiting line, his legs felt weak.

What would he say to his wife when he got home? This was the most difficult part. It would be even more disappointing for his sick wife to know that she had come so close to feasting on that fish. It would probably be best to tell her a lie. In all these many years of their marriage, it would be the first time that he had ever lied to her.

Seeing the old man standing there in a daze, one of the bystanders said to him, "You don't seem to know what goes on, do you? Before the foreign visitors come to look, they don't sell any of the good things. We all wait until they've come and gone before we hurry over to buy."

"You can buy them all right before the foreign visitors arrive," someone said sarcastically with a knowing air. "The only trouble is that you have to take them back. Last time, when Prince Sihanouk came to Nanking, they even brought in turkeys from somewhere. One of my neighbors had never seen a turkey, so, out of curiosity, he went and bought one. But he only got the turkey to the rear gate before it was sent back. They said they started with five turkeys, and after selling them for two days, there were still five turkeys!"

K'uai could not bear to listen anymore. He turned abruptly, and with a backward kick of his right leg, he mounted his bicycle.

"Comrade, he hasn't given you back the money yet!" some good-hearted person reminded him.

"He can give it to the foreign visitors!"

The old man spat fiercely on the ground as he shot another glance at the Tung Jen Street marketplace. Then he rode off without turning his head again.

* Chen Jo-Hsi 陳若曦, *Chenruoxi zi xuanji* 《陳若曦自選集》 (*Chen Rouxi: Selected Works*) (Taipei: Selected Works Press, 1976).

About the Editors

Jonathan Stalling is Professor of English and Curator of the Chinese Literature Translation Archive at the University of Oklahoma, where he is also Deputy Executive Director and a founding Editor of *Chinese Literature Today* journal and book series. Stalling is the author, translator, or editor of six books, including *Poetics of Emptiness* (Fordham), *Yíngēlìshī: Sinophonic English Poetry and Poetics* (Counterpath), and *Winter Sun: Poems,* by Shi Zhi (Oklahoma). Stalling's TEDx talks on Chinese-English interlanguage art and technology are available on YouTube; and his latest installation, "Poetics of Invention," can be found at https://poeticsofinvention.ou.edu.

Lin Tai-man 林黛嫚, born in Taiwan, holds an MA in Social Transformation Studies and a PhD in Chinese literature from Shih Hsin University. Former Editor in Chief of the Literary Supplement of the *Zhongyang ribao*《中央日報》(*Central Daily News*) and Editor of the *Renjian fubao*《人間福報》(*Merit Times*), she is now a full-time Assistant Professor of Chinese literature at Tamkang University in Taipei. Winner of many literary awards, including the Sun Yat-sen Literary Award, she has authored many volumes of essays, including *Shiguang migong*《時光迷宮》(*The Labyrinth of Time*) and *Ni daobie le ma?*《你道別了嗎?》(*Have You Bid Farewell?*).

Yanwing Leung 梁欣榮 holds a PhD in English and American literature from Texas A&M University and is currently Associate Professor of English at National Taiwan University, where he previously served as the Chair of Foreign Languages and Literatures and Director of the International Chinese Language Program. He is a poet and a translator who has taught writing and translation both at NTU and at the Ministry of Foreign Affairs, R.O.C. He practices traditional Chinese poetry in his spare time and is the author of *Lubai xin quan*《魯拜新詮》(*Poems Inspired by the Rubaiyat*) and *Lubai shiyi*《魯拜拾遺》(*The Forgotten*

Rubaiyat: A Verse Interpretation in Chinese). He is currently Editor in Chief of The Taipei Chinese PEN *Quarterly*.

CPSIA information can be obtained
at www.ICGtesting.com
Printed in the USA
FFHW021549131118
49382022-53685FF